SHOCK AND AWE
MUSCLE
BY TOM TYPINSKI

ISBN:

Published by TypinInc

Warren, Michigan

I would like to graciously thank the following for their contributions to this work:

Deborah Typinski *for all the photography created for this book.*

Thomas J. Typinski II *is the male model for the interior photos*

Fawn Gonyeau *is the female model for the interior photos*

Andrew and Heather Petrazsko *are the front cover models*

Keith Wurn *provided additional model photos in this second edition*

I would also like to graciously thank all the people who have been through this Shock And Awe Muscle System and have gotten great results, men and women, young and old. I have used it with teams, seniors, physically impaired, elite athletes and NPC/IFBB physique competitors. You are brave (and a little crazy!) Thank You.

TABLE OF CONTENTS

SHOCK AND AWE
MUSCLE BUILDING

Introduction

The system for this particular type of training is called "Shock and Awe." The 22 reps with a moderate weight provide the "SHOCK" to the muscles to pump them full of blood, prior to the "work" sets, the "AWE" sets of 11 reps.

Perform four sets total of 22, 11, 22, & 11 repetitions. The weight for 11 should be twice that of the 22 reps, i.e. 22 @ 60, 11@ 120. That is your ultimate goal. At first, gauging endurance will be tough. But you must get through the 22 reps, even if it takes 3 or 4 mini-breaks to get there. In time, not only will your stamina increase, but your strength will also increase to a level beyond where you began.

This method of "Shock and Awe" repetitions of 22/11, is fit for a man or woman, young or old. The "SHOCK" you supply is light enough to rehearse good form, but still challenging in the upper repetitions. The major focus should be in keeping perfect form from the first rep through to the last. The second and fourth sets will be difficult at first, as you will be struck by the "AWE" of weights you'd normally been able to handle; but you'll see poundages increasing by that 4th set every week. Strength planes upward as you train regularly with this method.

EXPERIMENT WITH SHOCK AND AWE MUSCLE

Apply "Shock and Awe" training to any bodypart, every exercise. First, use the ones outlined in this booklet, then try the methods on your own favorite movements and see how much more you get out of your workouts.

I suggest starting with one bodypart at a time; 3 exercises, 4 sets on one plane, 4 sets on another, then 3 high rep sets to finish off the bodypart, each with different weights, equipment and hand positions. Training 2 or 3 bodyparts at a workout will at first be insurmountable, even if that's what you're used to training.

The training must be done quickly, with very little rest between sets. Perfect form must be the main focus on every rep, every set. This allows you to cut deep grooves of separation between muscle groups and clean lines of execution over a full range of movement. The whole point is to avoid the "junkyard dog" approach of throwing weight around just to exercise your ego. Breaking the movement down to an almost isometric pace will be humbling. But the resulting muscularity will give a new impression to those watching, the "mere mortals" who dare not attempt sets over 10 reps; yes, those with the wraps around all their joints, looking more like parade day floats than healthy athletes.

The escalation of strength will have you back up to 110% of what you'd performed a month prior, as long as you stay true to the methods and repetitions.

WORKING COMPLEMENTARY MUSCLE GROUPS

The second component to "Shock and Awe" training is the compounded stimulation on a reversal of the movement, a complementary muscle group that is now working on the opposite side of the appendage. These are found in the Shock and Awe Supersets.

If you were arm training, you would work biceps and triceps alternatingly; both in a high rep warm up, then, with alternating sets of high rep biceps, low rep triceps, low rep biceps, high rep triceps and continue until 4 sets of each movement are accomplished, two of 22 and two of 11 reps, both exercises.

Change the angle, the exercise, the grip, and your muscles are now so pumped that you can barely go through the movements; but the weight is low and the form kept so strict, every single muscle fiber in both muscle groups are thoroughly saturated with blood, joints are filled with synnovial fluid and the arms contain a pump that's ready to tear the skin. And this isn't even halfway through the routine!

With isolation exercises, the muscle is trained but the surrounding support groups do not grow or work in synchronization with the whole body, therefore making the whole area only as strong as that one isolated muscle, and as weak as the weakest link. Use multiple joint exercises where the ankle, knee and hip; or wrist, elbow and shoulder are utilized; when power or strength are the goal.

The following Supersets are designed for the seasoned athlete. Do no jump right to these if you are just starting out. These are a goal to reach for later.

SUPERSETS

A superset means you go from one exercise to the next without rest. Do each of these supersets 4 times through, alternating 22 and 11 repetitions on each movement until two sets of 22 and two sets of 11 of each have been completed. The goal is to use half the weight at 22 that you use at 11 repetitions, sustaining or increasing with each successive set. If you are training for strength and size, add weight to the 11's; if you are training for endurance, add weight to the 22's.

CHEST-example:

22,11,22,11	Flat Bench Press	superset with
11,22,11,22	Decline Flyes	superset with
22,11,22,11	Dips	

LEGS-example

22,11,22,11	Walking Lunges	superset with
11,22,11,22	Squats	superset with
22,11,22,11	Extensions	

BACK-example

22,11,22,11	Pulldowns	superset with
11,22,11,22	Seated Pulley Rows	superset with
22,11,22,11	Barbell Rows	

TRICEPS-example

22,11,22,11	Close Grip Benches	superset with
11,22,11,22	Pushdowns	superset with
22,11,22,11	Kickbacks	

BICEPS-example

22,11,22,11	Barbell Curls	superset with
11,22,11,22	Dumbbell Curls	superset with
22,11,22,11	Cable Curls	

TRAINING DAYS:
2 days on (M,T)/ 1 day off(W)/
2 days on(TH,F)/ 2 days off(S,SU)

LEGS & SHOULDERS & CALVES - (Give yourself rest between leg and calf training)

BICEPS & TRICEPS & FOREARMS - (Give yourself rest between bicep and forearm training)

CHEST & BACK & ABS - (If abs are a priority bodypart, train them first in this group. They require the energy and focus.)

EATING SCHEDULE
Two days heavy protein/ very minimal carbs (Sat/Sun)
One day high carbs / moderate protein (M)
One day normal eating, low fat, moderate carbs (Tu)
Two days heavy protein, minimal carbs (W/Thur)
One day high carbs, / moderate protein (F)
One day normal eating, low fat, moderate carbs (Sat)
Two days heavy protein/very minimal carbs (Sun/Mon)

Eat your protein first, at every meal. Try to keep a steady stream of nutrients coming in at regular intervals. Never get too full, nor too famished. Eat every two to three hours maximum, and always be sure to search for the best possible foods. Keep fruit to a minimum but vegetables to a maximum, especially on high carb days. Most have essential calcium and magnesium necessary for recuperation and growth.

SHOCK AND AWE©

SHOCK AND AWE© - ABDOMINALS

There are different schools of thought regarding abdominal work. Do them fast and furious or slow and torturous, but do them. The three keys to any type of training regimen are attention, angles, and consistency. They are stubborn muscles and by attacking them -A,B,C - from Above the Belt, Below the Belt, and Across the Belt, you'll add greater depth and therefore better functionality and aesthetic appeal. The "Shock and Awe©"_approach requires high repetitions in successive, non-stop order across all three planes.

Your abdominals provide 70% of the support of your spine. They are your body's leverage point. Here are numerous variations of abdominal exercises, grouped according to the three primary methods of execution; lifting the legs, lifting the upper body, and crossing the midline of the body.

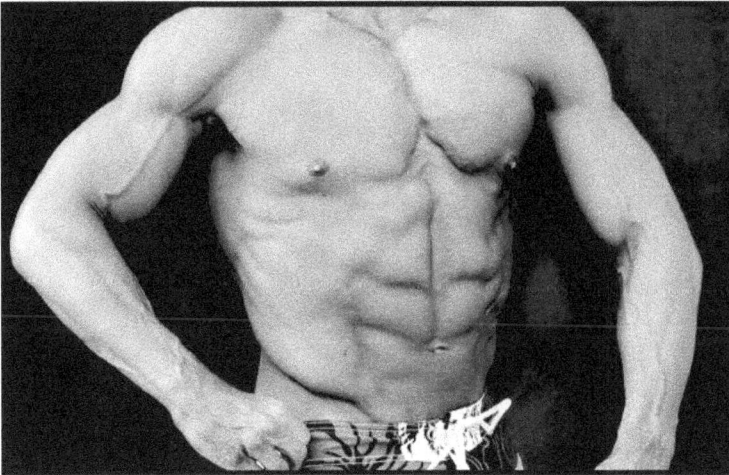

SHOCK AND AWE ABDOMINALS

These are the basic three movements to get you started.

ABOVE THE BELT

Crunch or Flat Back Sit-Up – The most common of all sit-ups moves.

Place both feet flat on the ground and draw the heels toward the butt. Place both hands behind the head and raise the upper body until the shoulder blades rise off the floor. The motion should cause you to exhale and draw the abs toward the floor, flattening the back and pressing the ribs downward. Do Not yank on the neck nor jerk the body up from the lower back.

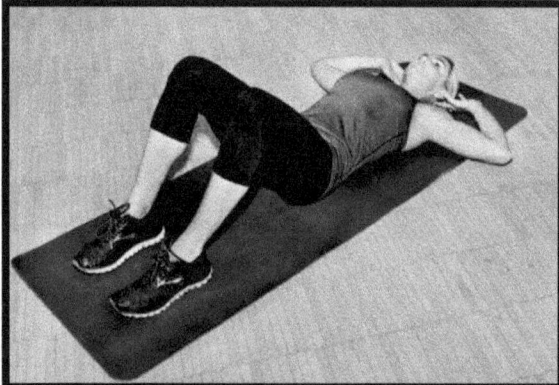

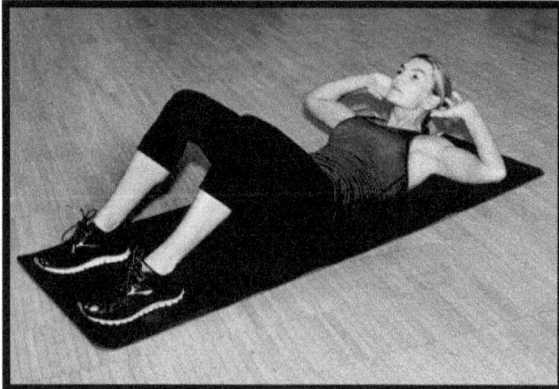

FLAT BACK SIT UP / CRUNCH

BELOW THE BELT

Leg Lifts – These can be done on the floor or on a bench with your legs hanging off.

Perform these with a slight bend in the knees and the lower back supported by placing the hands underneath the butt. Raise the head slightly to take further pressure off the lower back. Raise the legs high enough to pull the hips off the hands but be careful not to swing the legs up, but rather, bring

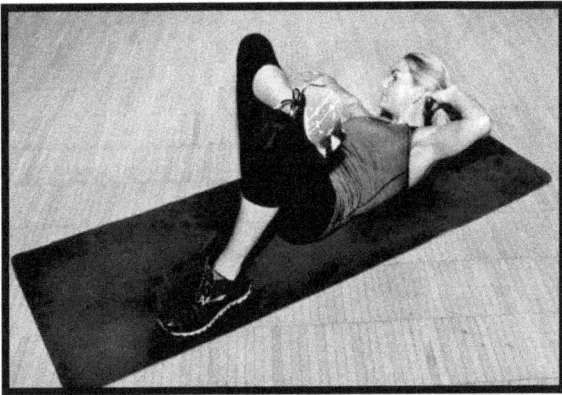

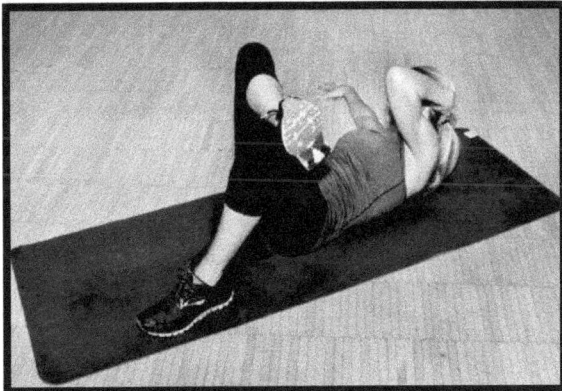

BENT LEG CROSSOVERS

them up with the abs. Lower them to the point of imprint, where the back lays flat on bench or floor.

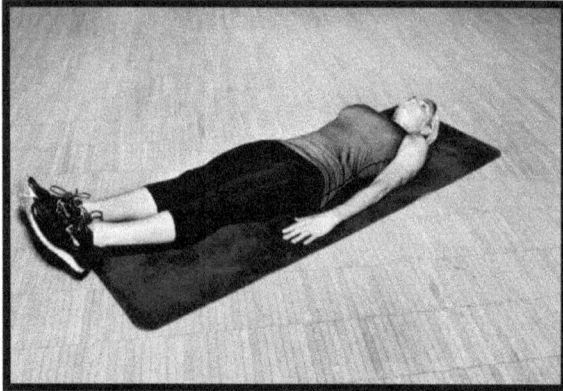

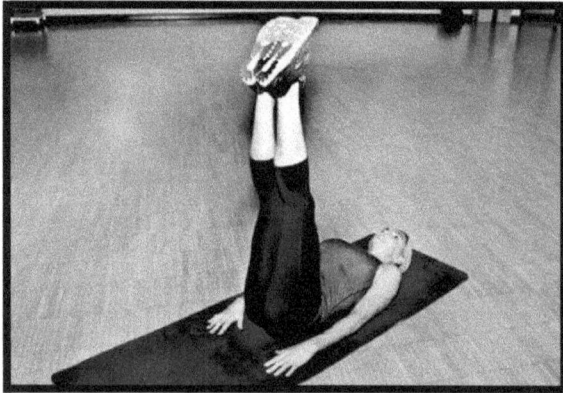

LEG LIFTS

CROSSOVER THE BELT

Bent Leg Crossover – From the Flat Back position, simply cross one foot over the opposite knee.

Ideally, both hands should be behind the head with the opposing elbow pivoted on the floor while the other elbow reaches to the opposite knee. Hitting all aspects of the abs consists of:

3 X 11-22 RAISING THE LEGS

3 X 11-22 RAISING THE BODY

3 X 11-22 RAISING AND TWISTING THE BODY ACROSS
      THE MIDLINE

Do the three movements in succession, then return to the first movement and begin your second set. At first, you may not get all 22 of each movement, just persevere and always get your reps.

Take 20 seconds or less breaks if necessary, but you'll see within 5 workouts that your endurance will escalate. Just be sure to do each movement as fully, with as much form, for every repetition, as possible. The misconception that the general public has with abdominal work is that they crunch to no end and wonder why their belly's are bunched up instead of flattened.

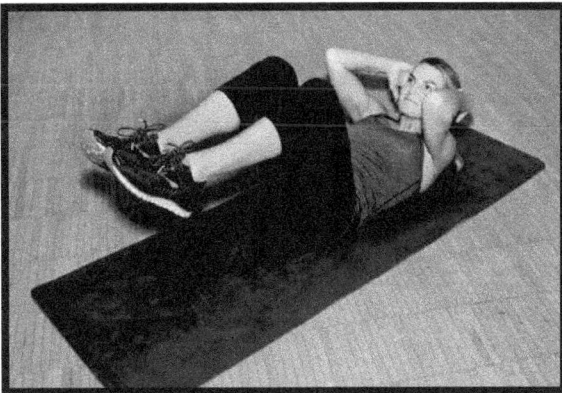

CRUNCHES WITH FEET UP

ABDOMINAL WORKOUTS

The reason there are more exercises for the lower Abdominals in these first groups, is that the lower abs often need the most attention and work, male and female.

#1 On Floor

        3 x 4 exercises moving from one to the next without rest

- 3 x 11 Leg Lifts – legs fully extended, raising feet until hips come off hands
- 3 x 22 Scissor Kicks – extending upper leg toward ceiling and lower, out and down
- 3 x 11 Crunches – regular gym class crunches with feet tucked toward butt, arms crossed over chest or holding back of head with elbows wide and gaze straight upward
- 3 x 22 Crossovers to Opposite Knee – sometimes called bicycles, but the legs should fully come in toward the opposite elbow, and extend fully away with toe pointed out, while the opposing elbow crosses to the contracting knee.

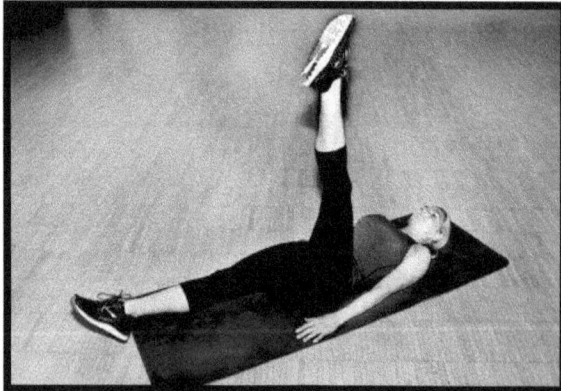

SCISSOR KICKS

It is important when doing these to work toward getting the outstretched leg fully extended so it's close to the ground and flattening out the abdominals. The lower abs get flat by extension, not by holding them in a contracted position. The arm must come fully across to touch the knee as well, to work the intracoastal muscles on the ribs. Keep the elbows wide to avoid pulling on the neck in this movement.

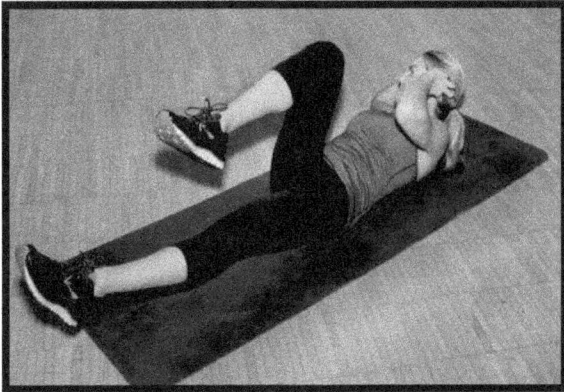

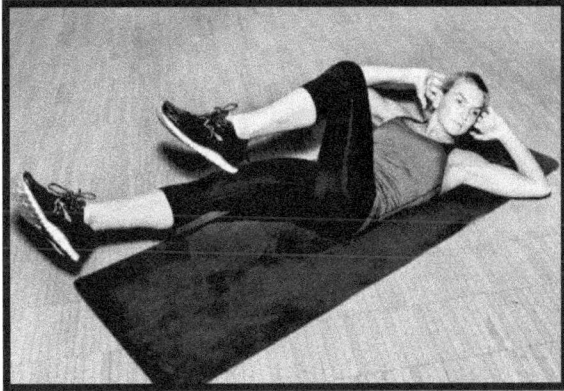

CROSSOVERS TO OPPOSITE KNEE

#2 On Floor

3 x 4 exercises moving from one to the next without rest

- 3 x 11 Pike ups – start flat on floor, lift arms and legs simultaneously to touch fingers to toes
- 3 x 22 Hand Slides – laying flat on back, raise legs 4 inches, slide hands along sides of body above the floor, toward the toes. Keep your feet raised and go to the next movement.

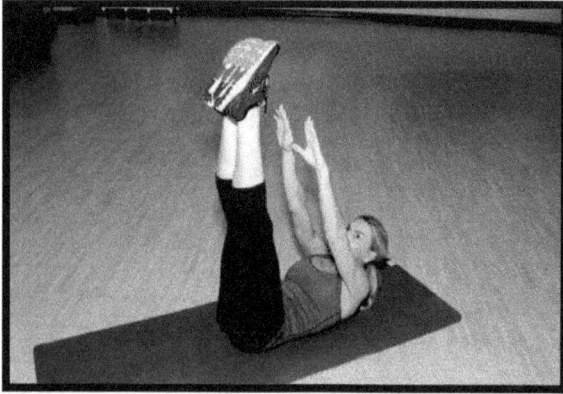

PIKE UPS

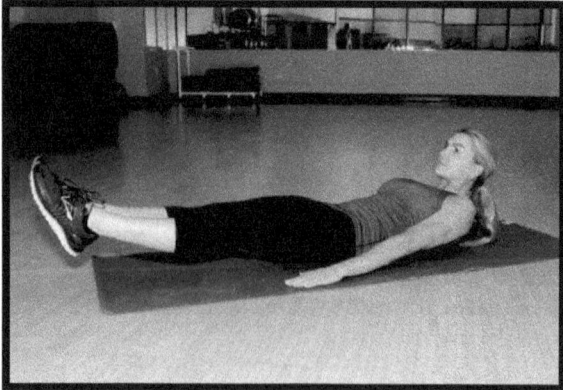

HAND SLIDES

- 3 x 11 Split Scissors – hands under buttocks, spread legs wide to sides, then back together, keeping head slightly lifted and chin tucked to chest.
- 3 x 22 Windshield Wipers – in 90° seated position, hands together in front of chest, twist to the left, touching fingertips to floor, then twist to right to touch floor, alternating until all repetitions are completed. Keep the back as straight as possible and hands high and pressed together as you twist.

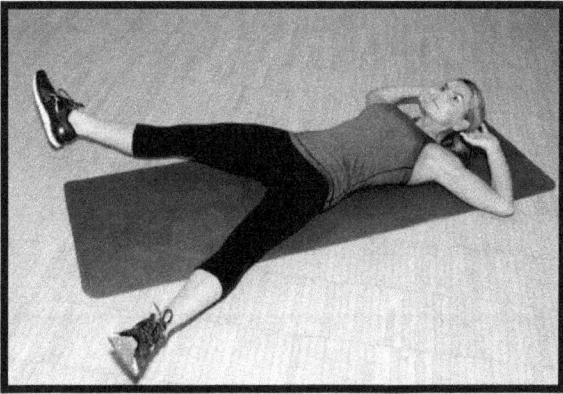

SPLIT SCISSORS

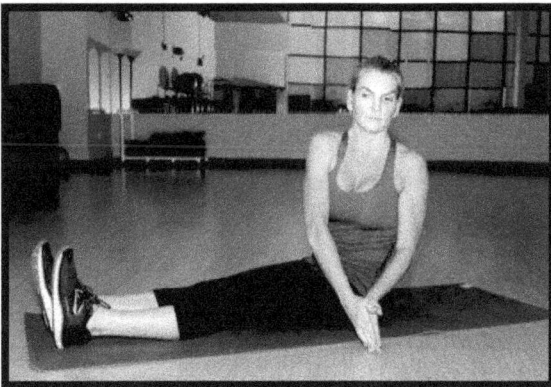

WINDSHIELD WIPES

The added resistance and balance required on a decline slant board trains more of the lower back, obliques and serratus as well as the abdominals. If you cannot do the previous routines well and completely - all sets, all reps, good form - do not begin these. There is a necessary progression of strength required and you have to earn the right to do these harder moves. Abs can be done daily and respond with consistent attention. One word of caution, adding weight to any abdominal move will make the muscle thicker and more prominent, just like every other muscle, so use weights minimally.

#3 On Decline Slant Board

- 3 x 11 Leg Lifts – feet toward the floor, hands on foot pegs, raise hips off bench as you get to the top of movement, pushing upward, not backward over head.

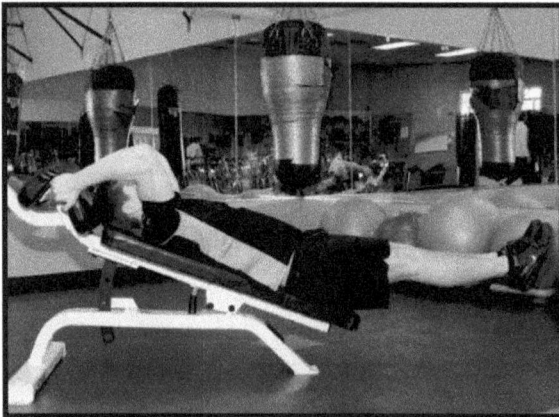

LEG LIFTS

- 3 x 22 Crossovers - elbow to opposite knee with shoulder blades brushing bench on rotation, crossing shoulder over mid-line of body, this stimulates serratus too.

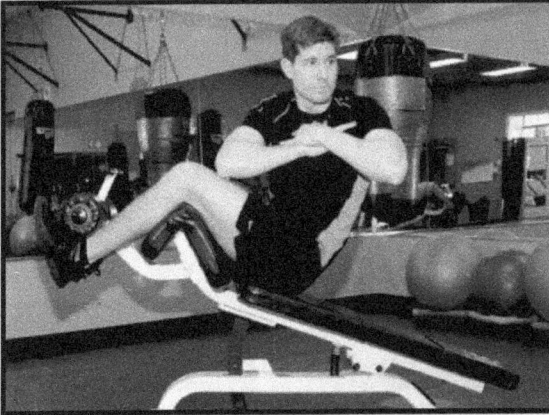

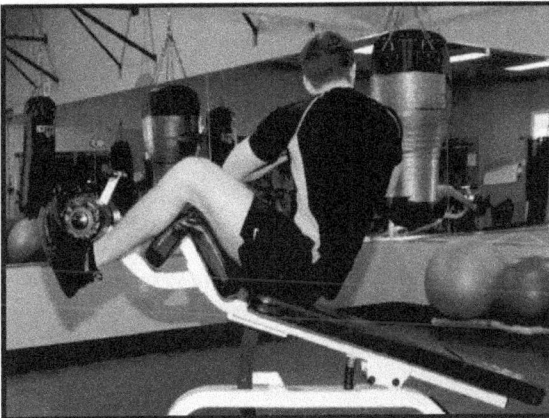

DECLINE CROSSOVERS

- 3 x 11 Weighted Sit-ups - arms folded across chest with 10 lb. plate/dumbbell; or holding medicine ball, hovering just over the navel, arms not contacting the body held lower to emphasize lower abs, higher for upper abs. It is important NOT to use too much weight to perform these Sit-Ups. The abdominal muscles, like any other muscle, grow thicker and bigger when you add weight to them. I would add as much form to them first, for added resistance, then add more sets, then more repetitions.

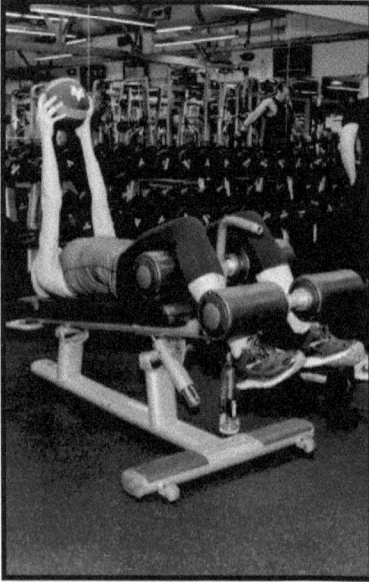

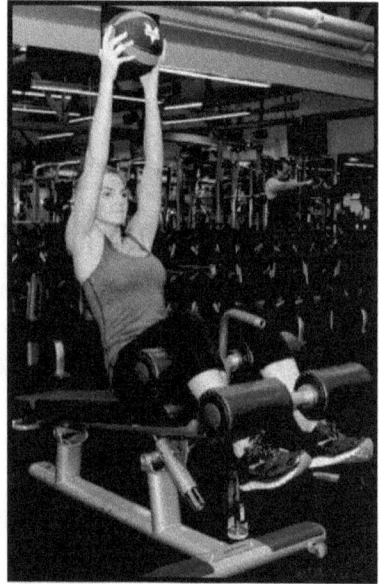

WEIGHTED DECLINE SIT-UPS

#4 On Decline Slant Board

• 3 x 11 Leg Lifts With A Kick - at top of movement, as hips roll up and off bench.

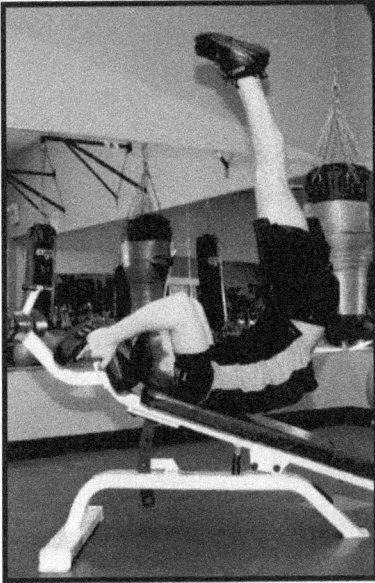

LEG LIFTS WITH KICK

• 3 x 22 Side-to-Side Touches or Serratus Steps in leaned-back position – keep body as straight up as possible with feet

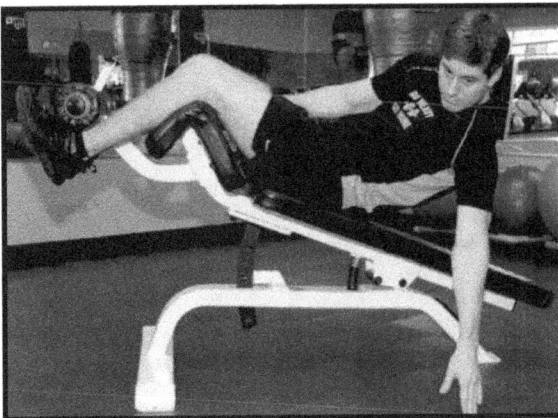

hooked on slant board. Lean left and right, touching floor on each side of bench without leaning back too far.

- 3x11"Keyholes"-with arms extended upward from a fully declined position, bring thumb and forefinger together over face into a triangular "keyhole", arms next to ears. Raise only shoulder-blades off board.

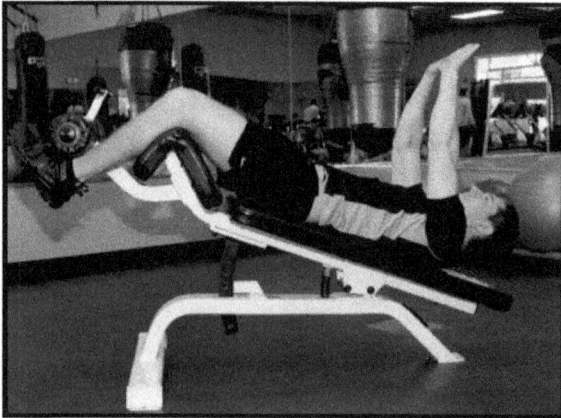

- 3 x 22 Straight Decline Sit-ups – full extension down, hard exhale at top of move.

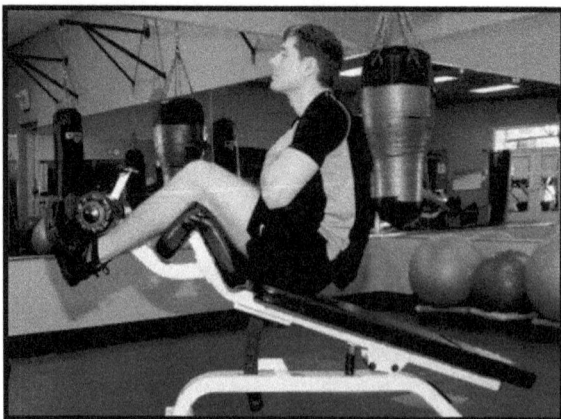

Make sure the Swiss Ball is the right height for your body. The taller you are, the higher the ball, usually in sizes from 55 – 75 cm. Be sure they are inflated enough to hold your weight, but not overinflated to the point where they throw you off on each bounce.

#5 With Physioball/ Swissball

- 3 x 11 Leg Lifts Holding Ball With Feet – hands under buttocks, legs straight out, raise until legs are perpendicular to the floor and hips rise slightly off the hands.
- 3 x 22 Bent Knee Swissball Touches – Begin with legs straight up, feet holding ball, with thighs perpendicular to torso. Bend at knees, lower ball toward floor, touch, return up.

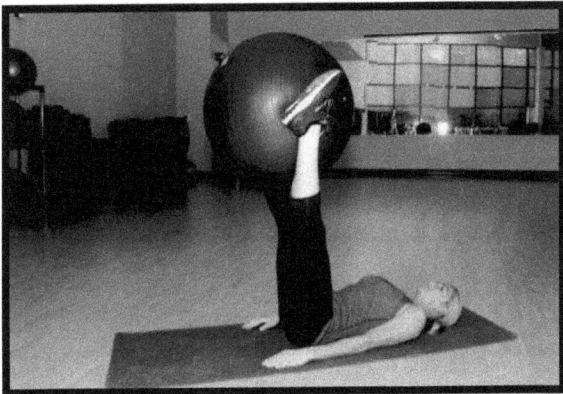

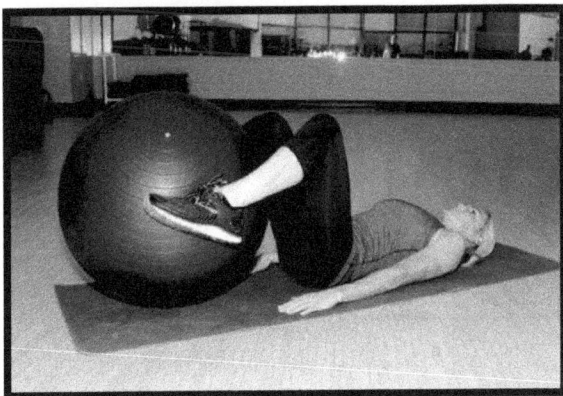

- 3 x 11 Planks with Ball Under Heels - arms out to sides, raise hips as high as possible   into a flat plank position. Touch tailbone to floor, raise hips back up to plank position.
- 3 x 22 Planks to Tucks to Crunches – Lay on floor, heels on ball, roll ball back toward glutes, raise upper body crunch-style with hands lightly on head and elbows wide and open. Return legs to straight position, fully lengthening abs and continue.

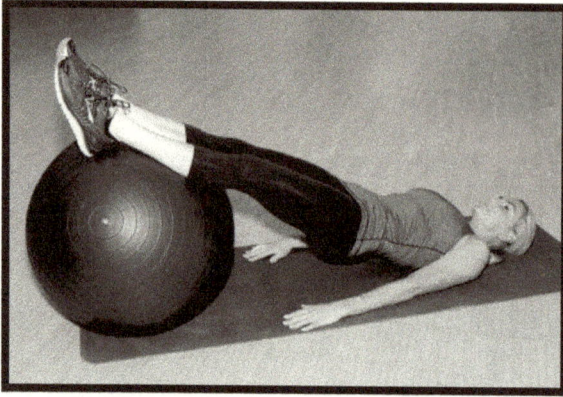

SWISSBALL PLANKS

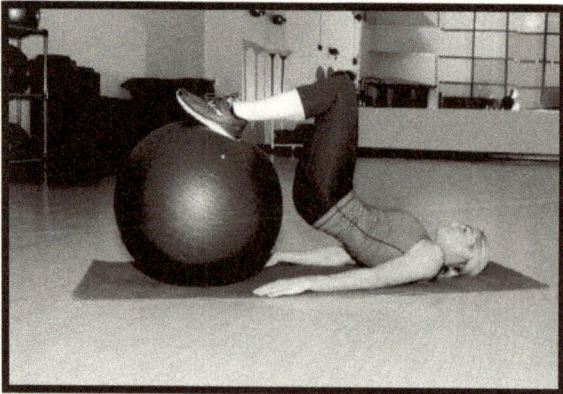

SWISSBALL CRUNCH

#6 With Physioball/ Swissball

- 3 x 22 Seated Crunches on Top of Ball – sit on the ball below center and crunch up
- 3 x 22 Crossover Crunches to Opposite Knee – just like regular crunches with a rotation

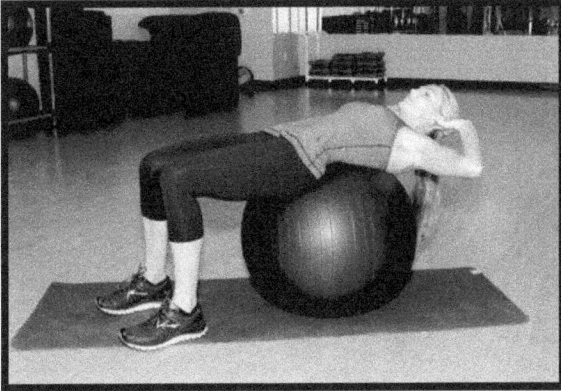

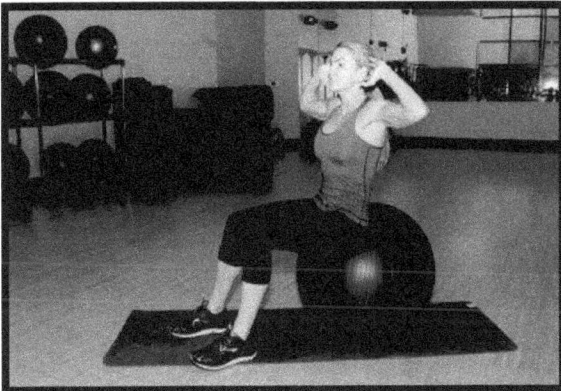

SEATED SWISS CRUNCH

17

• 3 x 11 Side Bends to each side – brace feet against wall, the side you're laying on is the foot that should be back, hip just below center of ball, hand on top hip, other hand lightly behind the head. Stretch body over ball and then rise up as high to side as possible.

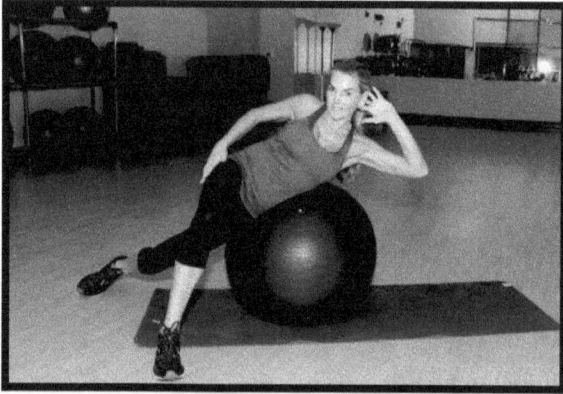

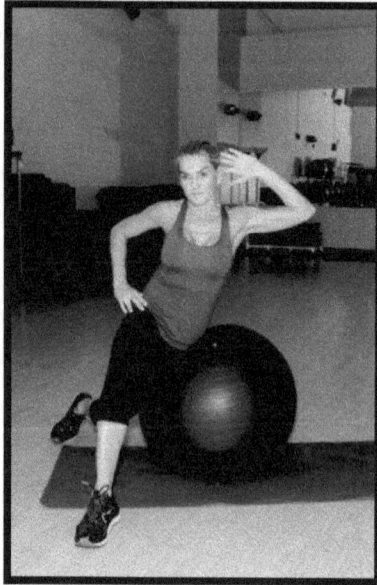

SIDE BENDS

ABDOMINALS/ SERRATUS/ OBLIQUES

This is my favorite abdominal combination for hitting the serratus, intercostals and obliques. The opposing gravities of lifting your legs from a hanging position, superset with weighted crunches on the floor from an overhead pulley, hits the upper and lower edges of the abdominals like no other combination. Remember, defining abs is about extending them completely, and contracting them forcefully, flattening, lengthening and holding them from as many angles as possible to give optimal depth and dimension.

By working opposing movements of pulling the legs up and then pulling weight down, gives the upper and lower ridges of the abs extra thickness, to stand out when your diet is tight. When doing them all the time in standard, flat positions, they lack the third dimension given when additional weight is used in a pull-down motion.

They must be done slowly, without jerking the body up or across the midline. Practice doing as many perfect repetitions as possible before worrying about getting all the reps. You will notice definition come in very soon as long as you are persistent and consistent.

#7 Hanging Leg Lifts With Arm Stirrups or Bar
superset with

- Weighted Pulley From Floor Position
- 11 Straight Hanging Leg Raises - from stirrups with legs
straight   *superset with*
- 33 Rope Pull Crunches To Knees - with full extension of abs at
top and full contraction and exhale at bottom.

The method for performing these is critical. The butt must sit on the heels and stay there throughout while the arms remain at 90° and the pull comes forcefully from the abdominals, not the back, the arms or the legs. Stay stationary and strict. Be sure to sit back on the heels fully, then to extend the ribcage while holding the arms stationary at the head; coming back down to a solid crunch, exhaling on the hold and drawing the abdominals toward the spine.

STRAIGHT HANGING LEG RAISES

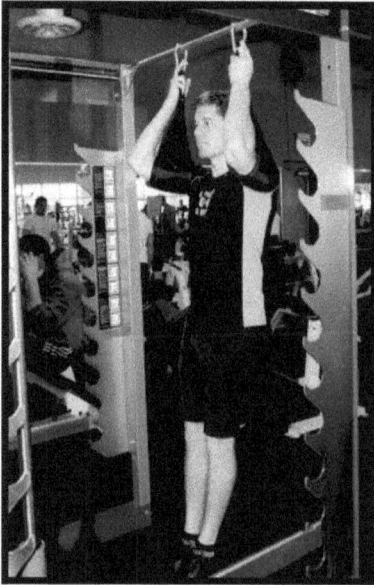

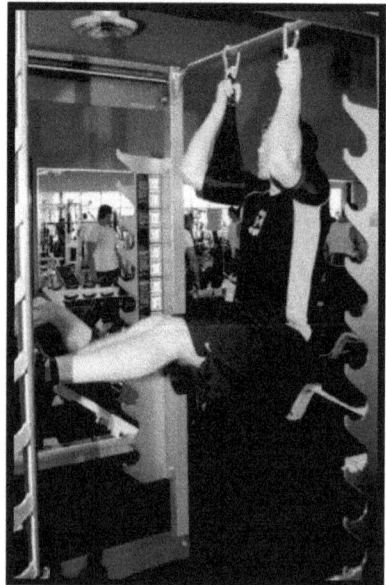

Do a vocal breath release to totally force the air out of your lungs and collapse your abdominals. The better you are able to control this movement by practicing here, the better you will be able to hold your abs in naturally, without thinking about it.

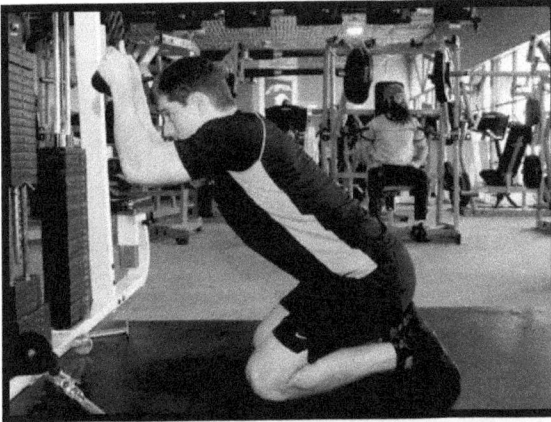

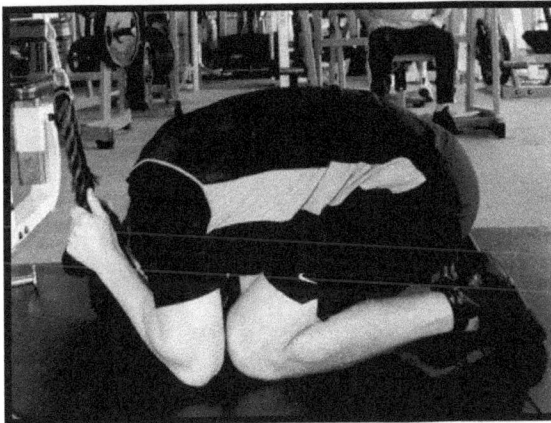

ROPE PULL CRUNCHES

• 22 Side To Side Hanging Knee-ups –The knees should rise up

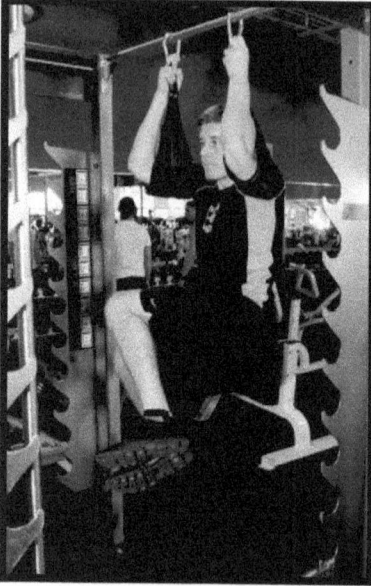

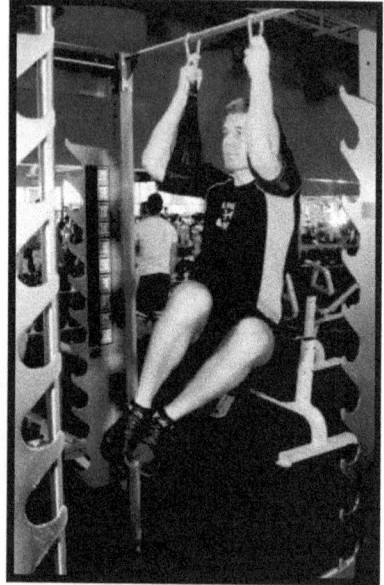

SIDE TO SIDE KNEE-UPS

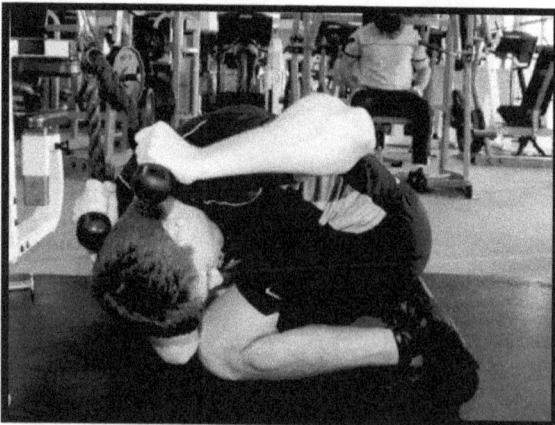

CROSSOVER ROPE PULLS

and to either side and high in center   *superset with*

• 22 Crossover Rope Pulls – Pull down, elbow to opposite knee, from same position on floor, only crossing over now to opposite sides on each alternation. Open the ribcage at the top.

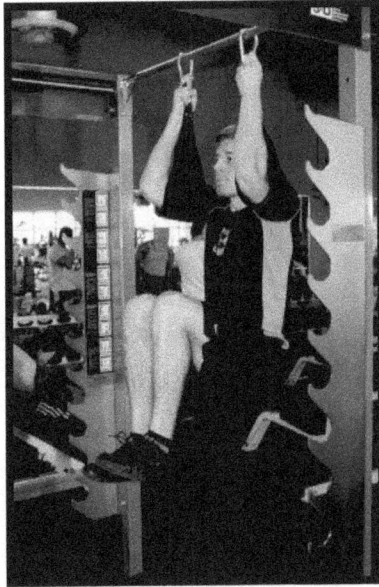

FRONT

LEFT

RIGHT

KNEE UPS

- 33 Front, Left, Right, Front Knee-ups - getting heels as high past hips as possible   *superset with*

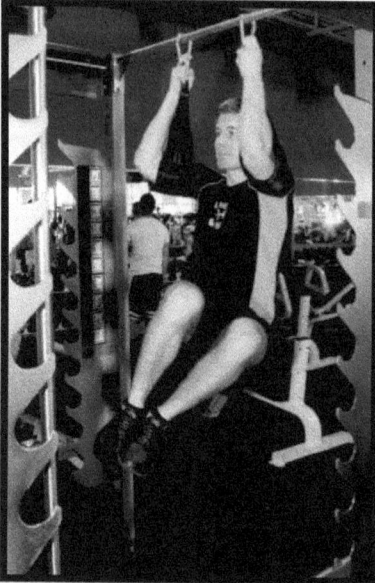

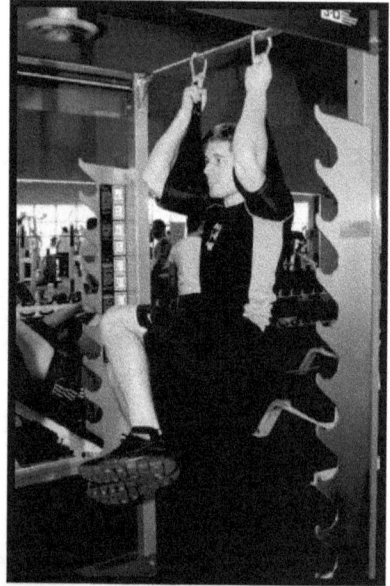

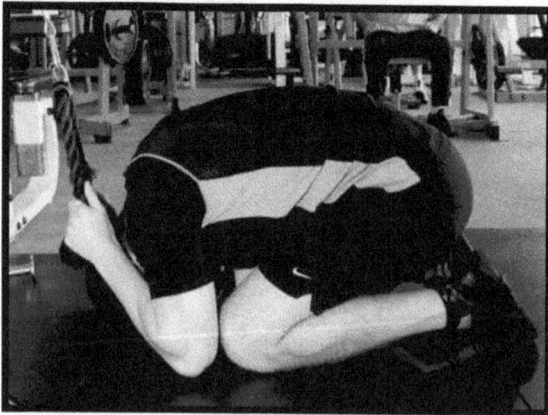

- 11 Heavily- weighted Rope Crunches - with squeeze-holds at bottom on exhale

CRUNCH VARIATIONS

These are unique in the fact that when the legs are raised upward, the lower abs are engaged; while raising the upper body activates the upper abs; and by crossing over the midline you also have the benefit of hitting the third, middle plane of abdominal training.

- 3 x 33 Feet Up Crunch – This can be done on a bench with a barbell across the uprights and the feet on the bar higher than the torso. It's important for you to rise up on your toes at the top crunch of this movement in order to "crunch" the upper and lower abs. Place your feet on the bar or edge of a bench, across the balls of your feet. As you pull up the torso toward the feet, pull the heels back toward the body so the lower abs crunch. Lay flat.

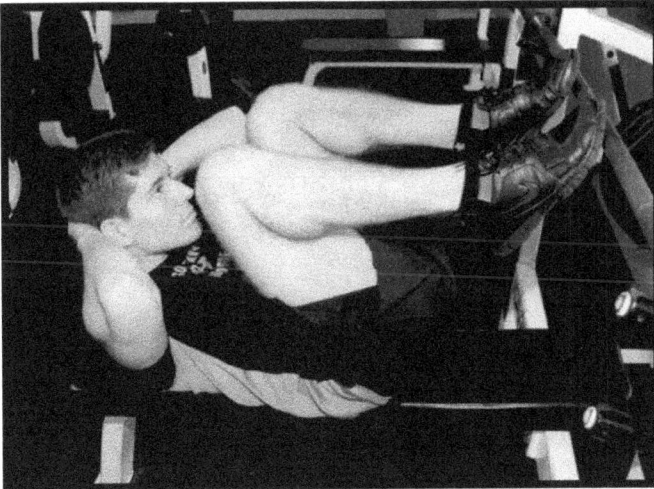

FEET UP CRUNCH

• 3 x 33 Heel Slide Crunch – The best way to do this is to lay on the floor with the heels across a bench or seat. As you pull your upper body up into its crunch, slide the heels back tight toward the torso while keeping them in contact with the bench. This is the tougher variation of the Feet Up Crunch and give your legs room to fully stretch at top.

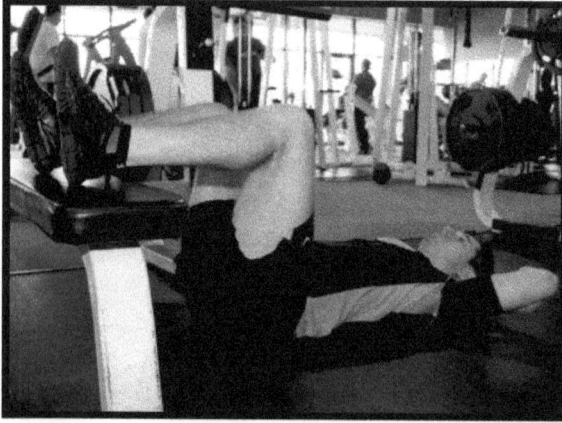

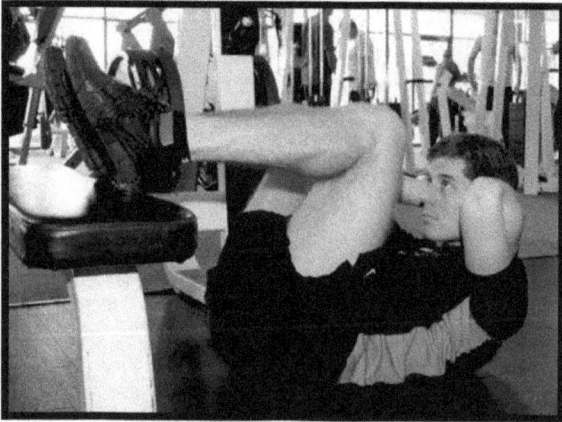

HEEL SLIDE CRUNCH

- 3 x 33 Pendulums – Hold the legs straight up 90° to torso, head off floor, arms out to sides initially for balance; roll legs to right, left, hold in center, then gently hold head and crunch to the middle, keeping the legs raised at 90° the entire set.

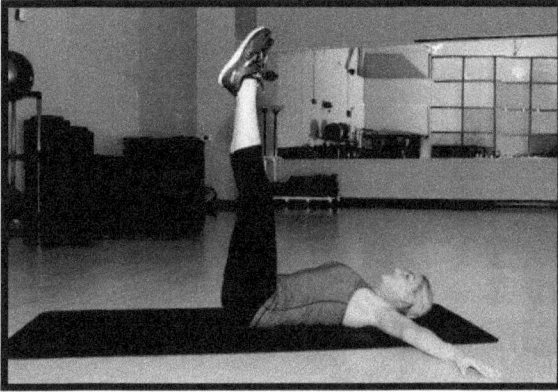

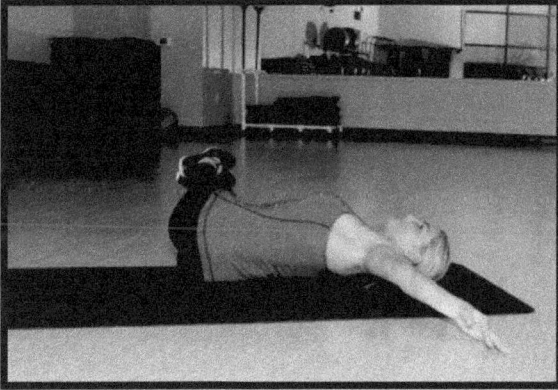

PENDULUMS

- 3 x 33 Pike Crunches – raise legs straight up, reach arms to left, right and center, "1,2,3" until 33 total. On an advanced level, do the same with a medicine ball in hands.

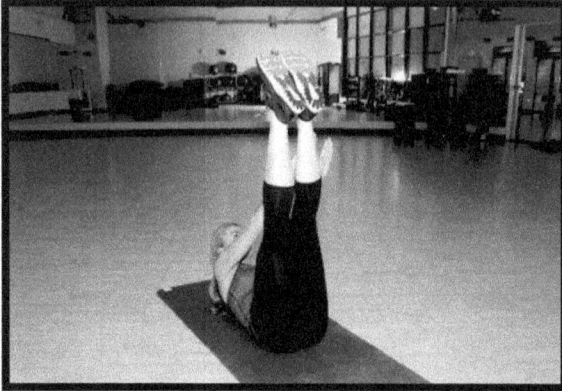

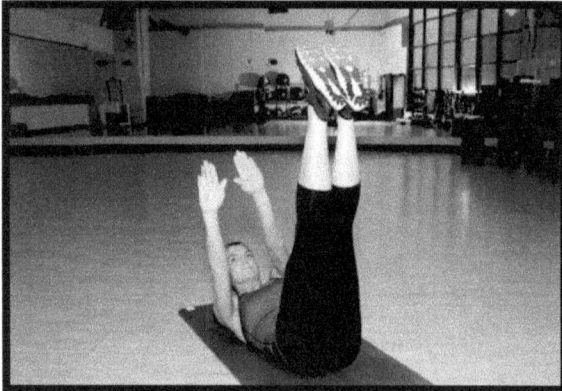

Left, Center, Right
PIKE CRUNCHES

- 3 x 22 Upper Ab Reaches – place heels on bench, legs bent at knees 90°, stretch arms completely overhead, reach back, then forward and up.

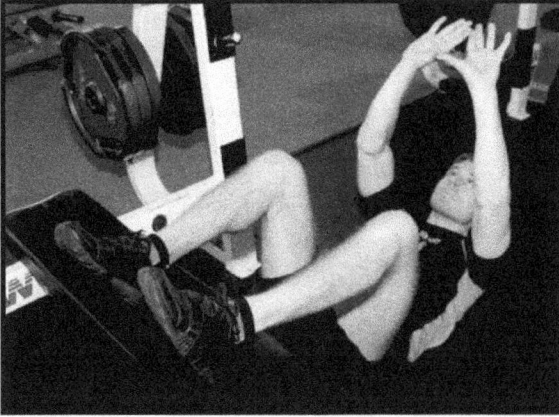

Additional BELOW THE BELT Abdominal Exercises:

- Scissor kicks - Do these laying flat on the floor, with the hands under the butt supporting the back.

Kick the legs apart and reach for the ceiling with toes pointed on the upward leg, while consciously pulling the lower leg toward the floor. Do not let the legs flail by bending too much at the knees, keep them strict and pull in both directions from the abdominals.

- Deep Breaths – Draw breath in for 4 counts, hold for 7, exhale for 8, fully releasing while simultaneously drawing the navel toward the spine. Hold it in and draw a second breath. These are also known as "vacuums" when you continue holding in while inhaling and exhaling and are bent at the waist 90° with the face parallel to the floor.

- Single Leg Scissor Kicks – Begin these by laying flat on the floor. Raise one leg up straight until the other comes off floor 6 inches, hold for a count of 3, then slowly lower and alternate the legs to complete a set of 22, or 11 per leg. Do not let the legs pass each other, bring all the way to the top, return to the bottom, then repeat with other leg.

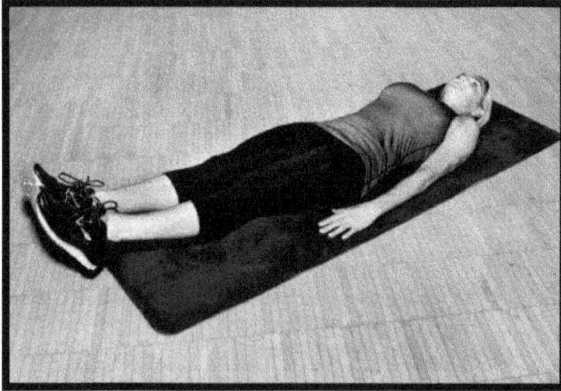

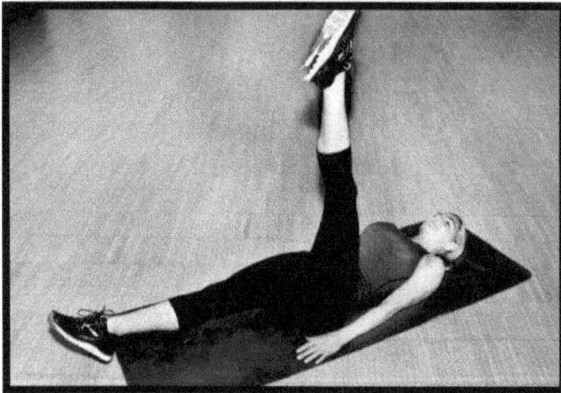

SINGLE LEG SCISSOR KICKS

SHOCK AND AWE © SUPERSETS - ARMS

These are not to be confused with straight Shock And Awe sets for either the Biceps or the Triceps. You can take any one of these workouts and concentrate exclusively on one or the other, but these were designed with true Shock And Awe in mind, to hit opposing muscle groups with no rest in between.

The final one is the Ultimate Shock And Awe Arm Superset and is comprised of what I call parts A & B, each part consisting of 4 exercises.

On the A you move through 4 sets of Triceps, then go to 4 sets of Biceps and continue alternating between the two muscle groups. These are best done with a partner, so the only rest you'd get is when they're doing their set.

The second part, B, consists of 2 Biceps and 2 Triceps moves and you literally go nonstop between all 4 in alternating fashions of 22 and 11's until all 16 sets are complete. This is "The Monster In The Closet" workout. This will tear up any mere mortal. I suggest you work your way through the earlier workouts and attempt this after a month of the other Shock And Awe Supersets.

I've included the number of sets and reps comprised in each workout. The secret here, in a word, is, <u>VOLUME</u>. By pumping so much blood volume through your muscles in this fashion over two bodyparts, you cannot touch the amount of pump you get out of a workout in comparison to these Shock And Awe sessions. It just makes so much sense to be able to gauge your exercises and set your goals according to 22 repetitions in slow, strict warm-ups, followed by an 80-90% work-set at twice the weight, then back to a second pumping set at 11% more, and finishing off with a fourth set at near maximum for 11 repetitions.

Choose your favorite workout and give me feedback at: www.shockandawemuscle.com.

SEE YOU IN THE GYM!

#1 BICEPS & TRICEPS

(On your way to not so "merely mortal")

(25 sets/ 726 reps)

• 4 x 22-11 Close Grip Bench Press – hands as close as comfortable, let elbows flare to sides

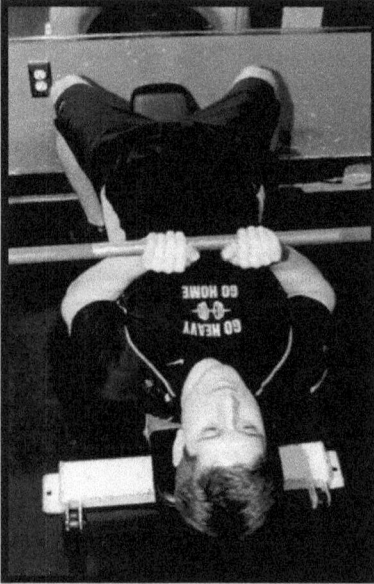

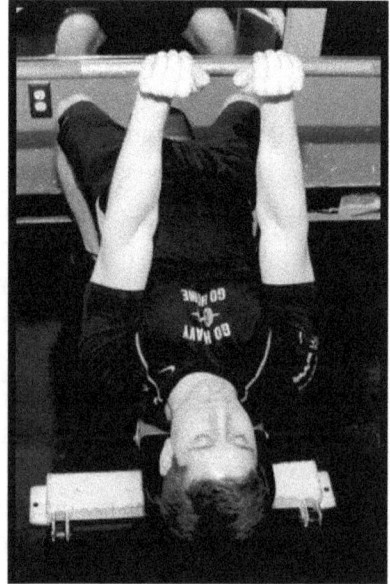

CLOSE GRIP BENCH PRESS

Hold your hands as close as possible without compromising the wrists, with the thumbs under the bar. Let the elbows flare at the bottom of the movement, to incorporate the large, long head of the Triceps, as well as the medial and outer heads. This is an overall strength building move in addition to an essential Triceps exercise.

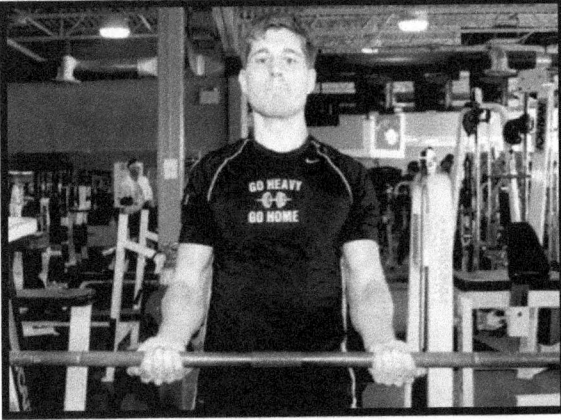

*BARBELL
CURLS*

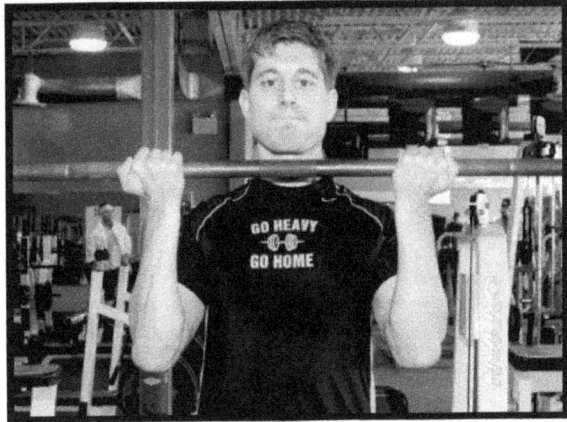

- 4 x 22-11 Barbell Curls w/Straight Bar – thumbs tucked in
  "Monkey Grip" under bar

By holding your thumbs under the bar in this manner, you force the stress to the outer, lower portion of the Biceps; thus, giving it a fuller and more rounded insertion at the elbow.

- 4 x 22-11 Overhead Rope Triceps Pulls – elbows in and high, pushing straight forward; if you're hitting your head, your elbows are too low, or your head too high.

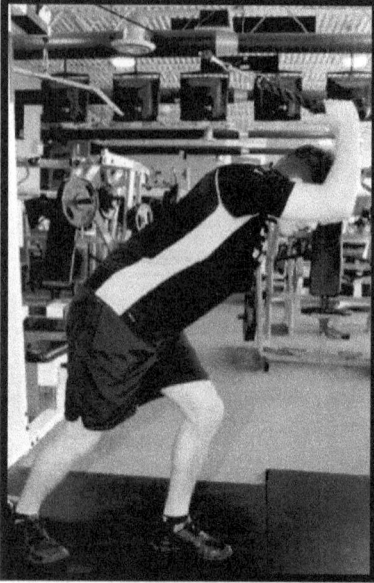

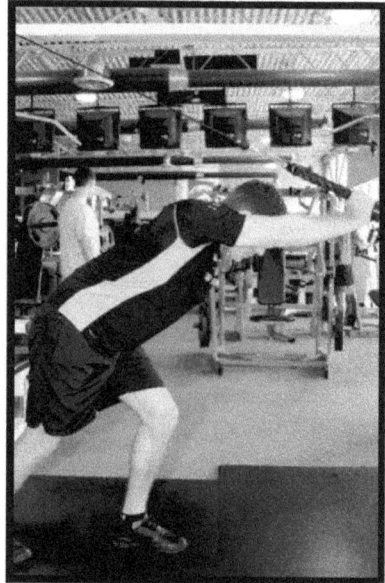

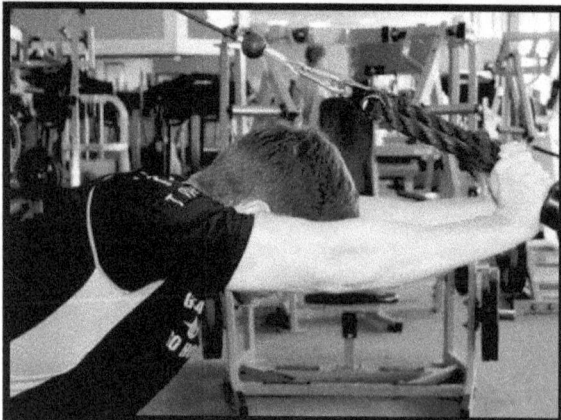

TRICEPS OVERHEAD ROPE PULL

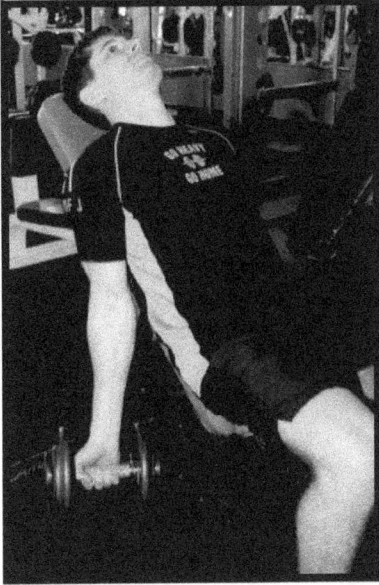

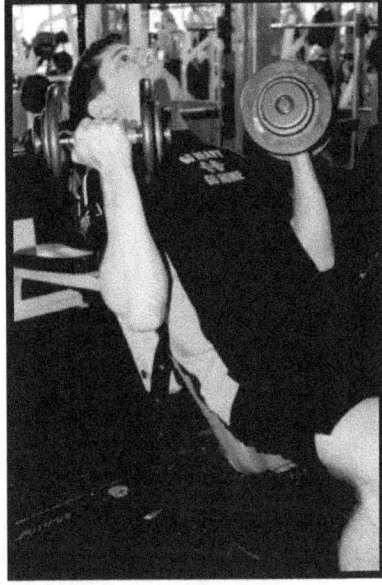

SEATED INCLINE DUMBBELL CURLS

- 4 x 22-11 Seated Incline Dumbbell Curls - It is important to let the arms hang down fully at the bottom, the head to rest against the bench, and the elbows to stay low as you pull fully through the biceps and not lift through the shoulders.

Mini B - Giant Superset To Finish (If you dare!)

• 3 x 22 Triceps Pushdowns – back straight, chin up, shoulders down and back, arms 90° at top; push and hold at bottom of movement to really "burn in" the definition of the Triceps muscles.

*DO NOT LEAN OVER THE BAR, MAKING THE HEAD, NECK AND TRAPEZIUS BECOME INVOLVED IN THE MOVEMENT. THIS TAKES THE STRESS OFF THE TRICEPS AND ONTO THE SHOULDERS.

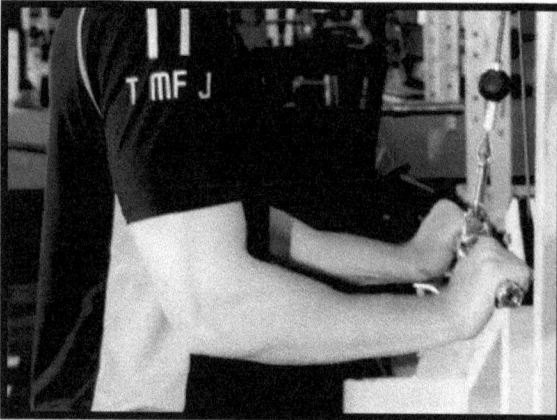

TRICEPS PRESSDOWNS

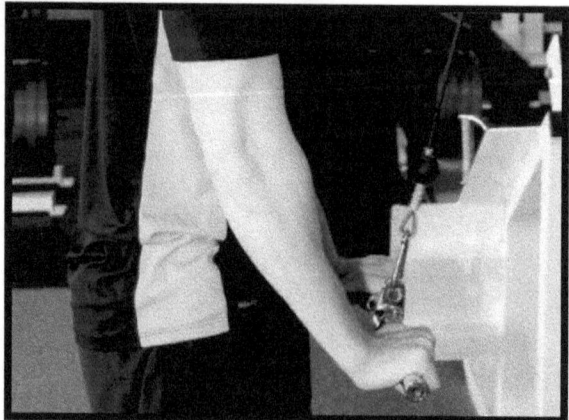

• 3 x 22 Triceps Rope Pulldowns – keep hands together on rope, do not pull to sides, roll small finger out and up while holding the thumbs together.

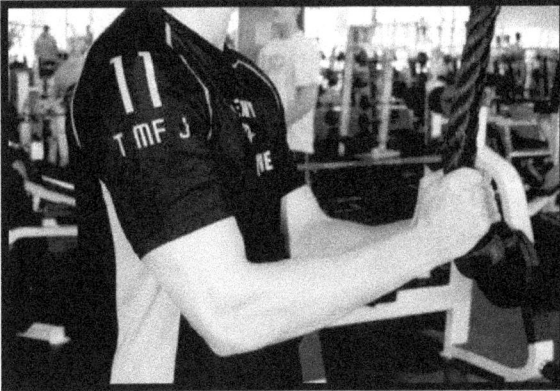

**TRICEPS
ROPE
PULL
DOWNS**

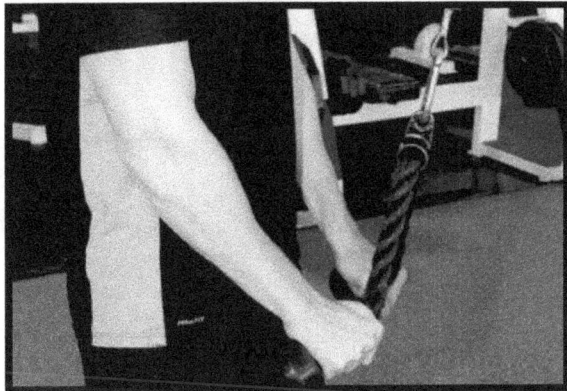

This allows the inner portion of the Triceps insertion at the elbow to become defined. Pressdowns with the bar accentuate the outer head. If you use too much weight here and pull the handles out to the sides, you incorporate the middle head of the Triceps, which shows predominantly on the outside of the arm.

• 3 x 22 Seated Pulley Curls – with a short handle on a pulley-row machine, and elbows at sides, reach forward without raising the arms too high; then, keep the elbows low on the curl with the wrists forced toward the body, to stress the "Peak" of the Biceps. The arms should remain stationary throughout, rather than any up/down, or forward and back movement.

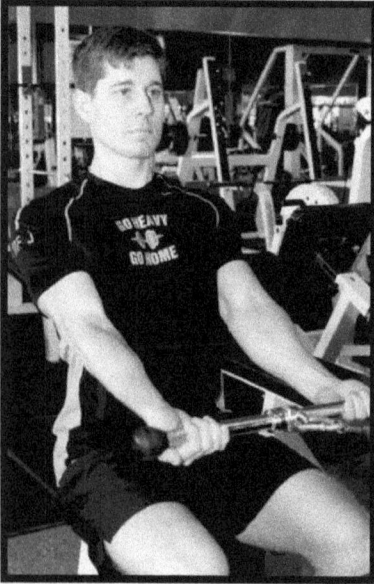

SEATED
PULLEY
CURLS

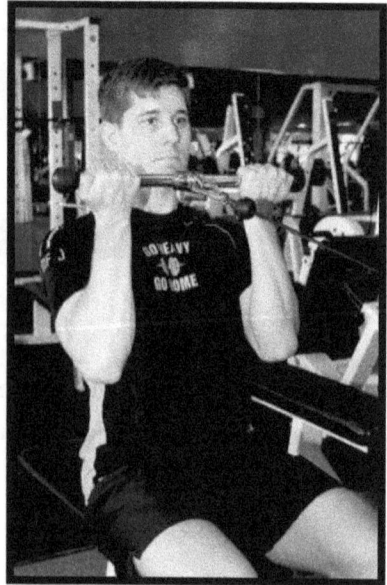

#2 BICEPS & TRICEPS
(23 sets/ 418 reps)

- 3 x 22 Close Grip Bench Press   *superset with*
- 3 x 22 Standing Barbell Curls

- 4 x 11 Overhead Triceps Rope Pulls – Heavy
- 4 x 11 Straight Bar Preacher Curls - Heavy

- 3 x 22 Triceps Pressdowns   *superset with*
- 3 x 22 Triceps Rope Pulls   *superset with*
- 3 x 22 Close Grip Cable Curls

Rest only after completing whole set of 3 movements, no stops, just weight drops, in between.

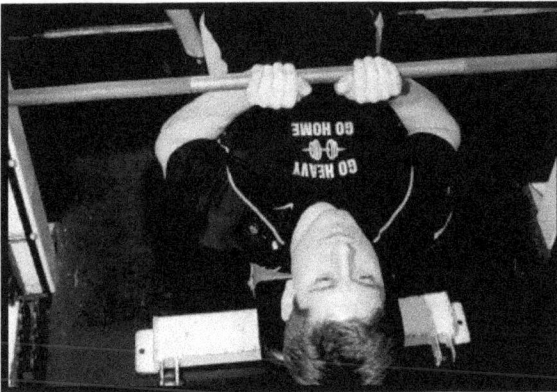

CLOSE GRIP BENCH PRESS

#3 BICEPS & TRICEPS
(23 sets/ 396 reps)

- 4 x 22 -11 Close Grip Bench Press
- 4 x 22 -11 Barbell Curls
- 4 x 22 -11 Overhead Rope Pulls
- 11, 11, 11, 33 Barbell Preacher Curls – add weight first 3 sets, then drop incrementally last set

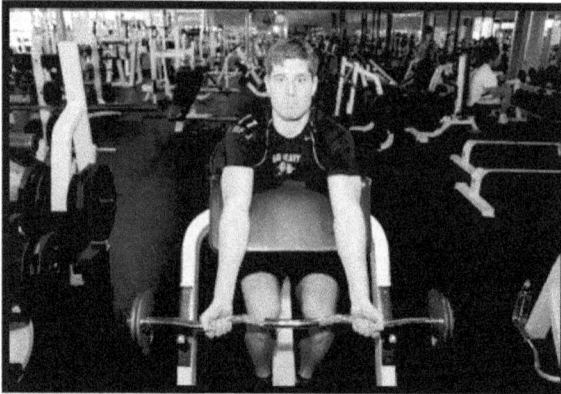

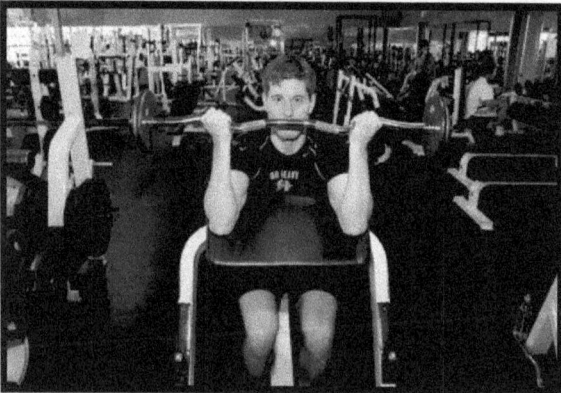

BARBELL PREACHER CURLS

- 3 x 22 Front Rope Pushdowns
- 4 x 22 Alternating Dumbbell Curls – with twist at top over biceps head, inner bell rotates over bicep   superset with
- 11 Throwbacks – elbows stay stationary on hips, curl toward the outside at the biceps-brachialas tie-in to target the lower-outer biceps

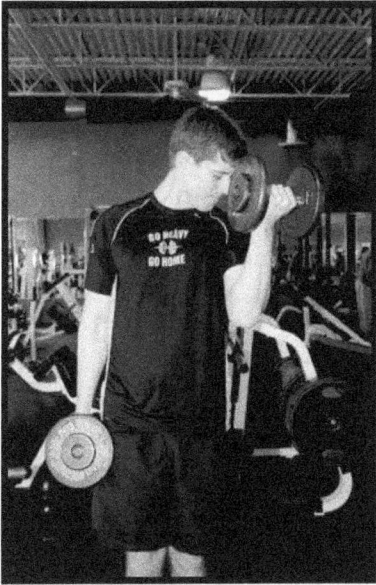

ALTERNATING CURLS

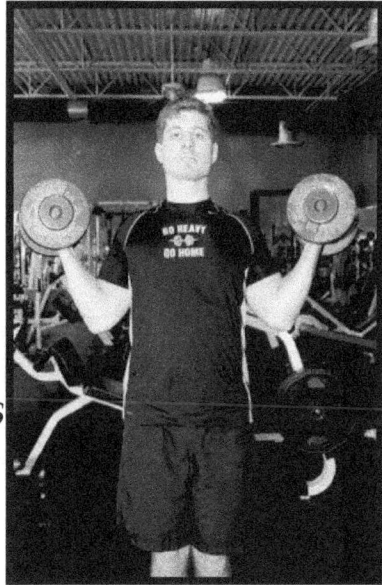

DUMBBELL THROWBACKS

41

#4 BICEPS & TRICEPS (Biceps Priority)
(32 sets/484 reps)

- 4 x 22-11 Straight Bar Curls
- 4 x 22-11 Decline Skull Crushers

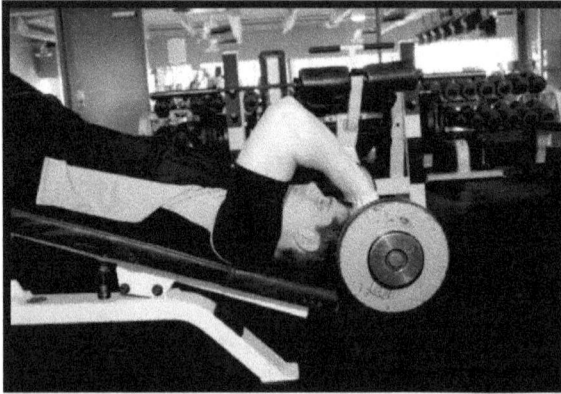

DECLINE SKULL CRUSHERS

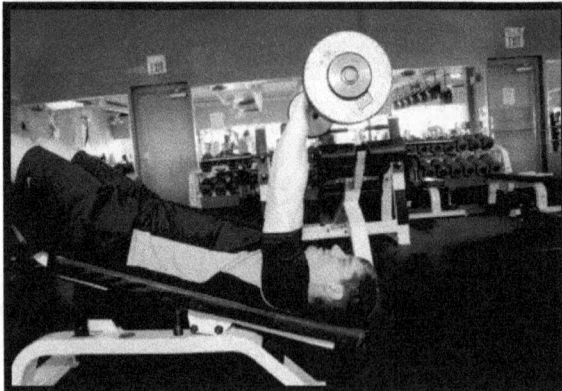

The Skull Crushers are best done with an E-Z Curl bar and should drop just over the forehead, not to it; with elbows held in tight and pointing straight up.

- 4 x 22-11 Incline Dumbbell Curls
- 4 x 22-11 Overhead Rope Pulls

- 4 x 11 Single Handle Curls   *superset with*
- 4 x 11 Single Handle Reverse Triceps Pulldown

- 4 x 22-11 Close Grip Preacher Curls
- 4 x 22-11 Close Grip Bench Press

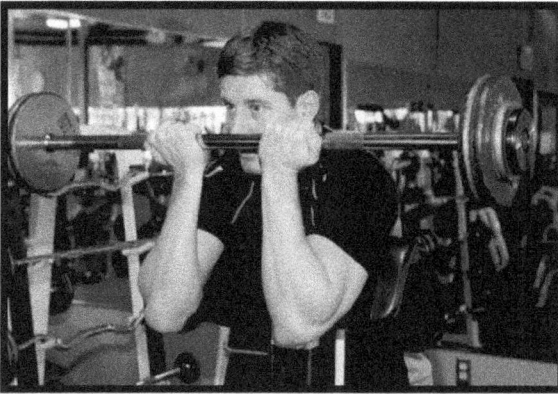

CLOSE GRIP PREACHER CURLS

The close grip on these last two exercises forces the stress to the center of the muscles; the peak on the biceps and the long head of the triceps.

It is important to do these exercises in the prescribed order. Once you become accustomed to Shock And Awe Training, you can try out your own favorite movements and adapt the workouts accordingly. If supersets are not highlighted, do the whole exercise all the way through to completion. These variables are all part of The System.

#5 BICEPS & TRICEPS (Triceps Priority)
(25 sets / 462 reps)

- 4 x 22-11 Close Grip Bench Press   *superset with*
- 4 x 22-11 Standing Barbell Curls

- 4 x 22-11 Overhead Rope Triceps   *superset with*
- 4 x 22-11 Incline Dumbbell Curls Together

- 3 x 22 Triceps Pushdowns   *superset with*
- 3 x 22 Triceps Rope Pulldowns   *superset with*
- 3 x 22 Seated Pulley Curls

#6 BICEPS / TRICEPS / FOREARMS
(33 sets / 473reps)

Biceps

- 3x 22 Standing Alternate Dumbbell Curls superset with
- 3 x 22 Preacher Straight Bar Curls   *superset with*
- 3 x 11 Heavy E-Z Bar Curls

Triceps

- 4 x 22-11 Close Grip Bench Press   *superset with*
- 4 x 11 Overhead Ropes   *superset with*
- 4 x 22 Pushdowns

Forearms

- 4 x 11 Reverse Curls   *superset with*
- 4 x 11 Zottman Curls   *superset with*
- 4 x 22 Wrist Curls

#7 SHOULDERS / TRICEPS / BICEPS
(30 sets / 495 reps)

Shoulders

- 4 x 22-11 Barbell Shoulder Press on Smith
- 3 x 22 Rear Deltoid Cable Pulls   *superset with*

• 3 x 11 Cable Side Laterals

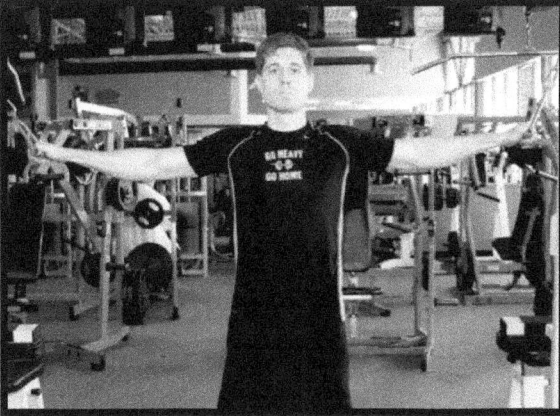

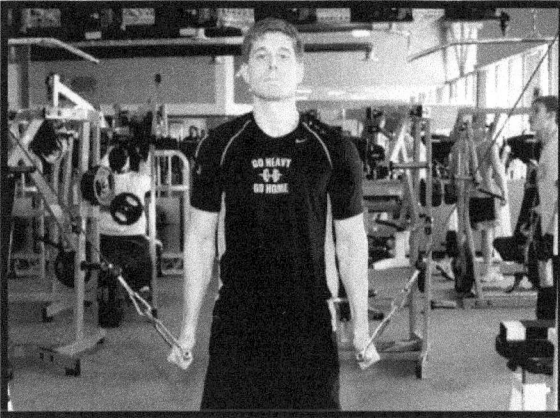

CABLE SIDE LATERALS

Triceps
• 4 x 22-11 Close Grip Benches
• 3 x 22 Triceps Pressdowns   *superset with*
• 3 x 11 Overhead Rope Pulls

Biceps
- 4 x 22-11 Barbell Curls
- 3 x 22 Dumbbell Incline Curls   *superset with*
- 3 x 11 Dumbbell Concentration Curls

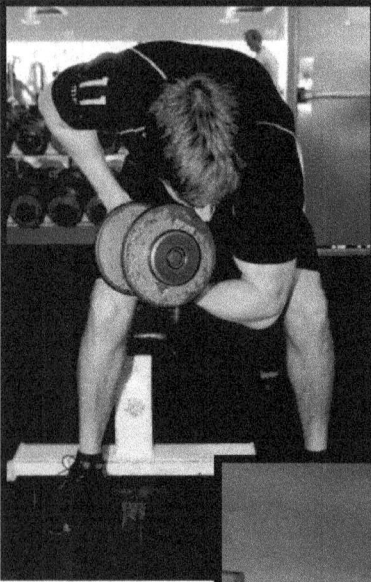

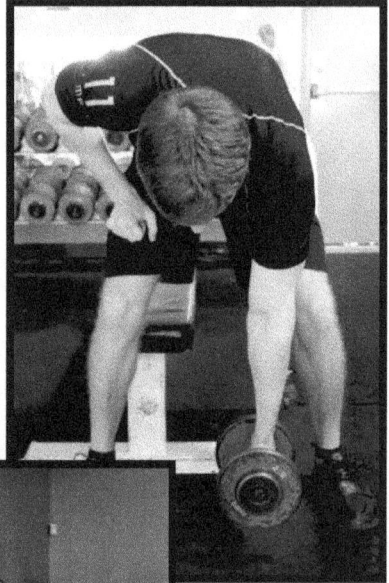

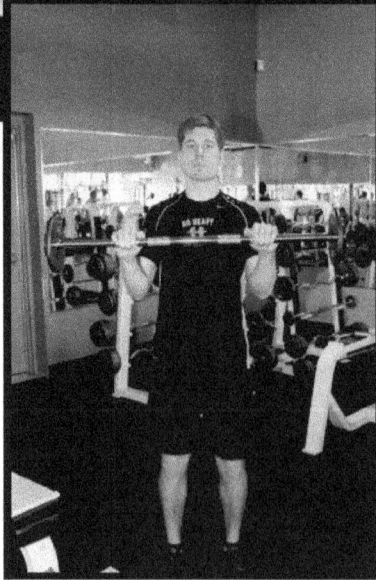

REVERSE CURLS

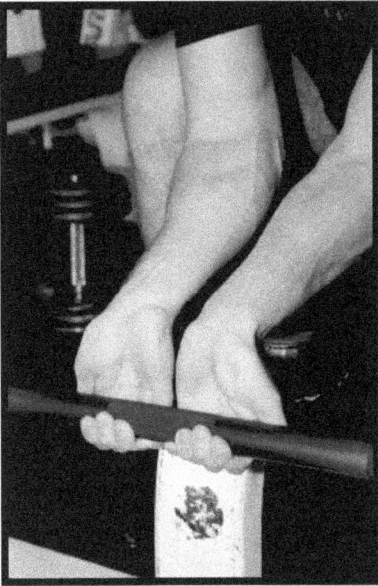 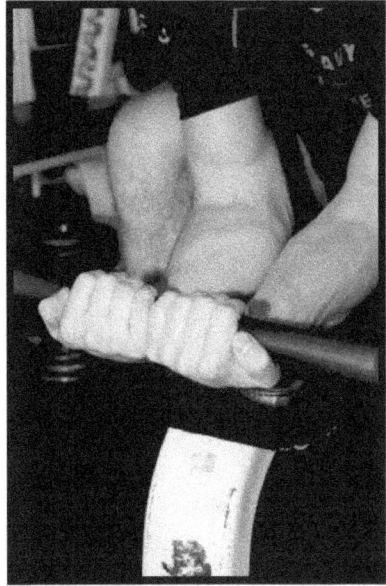

WRIST CURLS

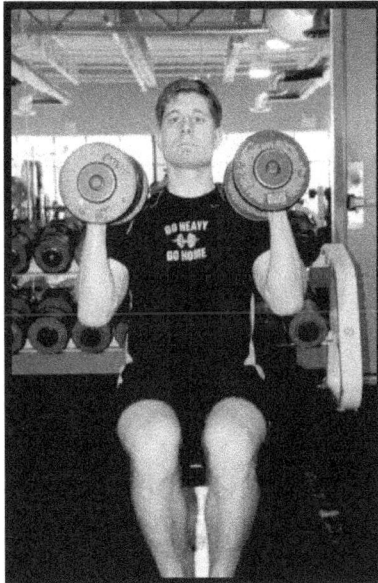

ZOTTMAN CURLS

CAUTION: EXTREMELY ADVANCED WORKOUTS

The following workouts, 8, 9, 10, 11 and The Monster are very high volume workouts. Not that the previous workouts of nearly 500 repetitions were not! Do not try to go directly to these workouts before your body is ready for them. Do at least a month of the first 7 workouts to adapt your endurance to the volume created. You may find the first 7 sufficient, but I guarantee there will be a time when you're up for a greater challenge and these last four workouts will satisfy the need. And above all, remember, it's the form, not the weight, which creates the shape of the muscles, so stay strict.

#8 BICEPS & TRICEPS
(37 sets/ 539 reps)

- 3 x 22 Standing Alternating Curls *superset with*
- 3 x 11 Dumbbell Throwbacks

- 4 x 22-11 Decline Skull Crushers *superset with*
- 3 x 22 Dips

- 4 x 22-11 Low Throwback Curls
- 4 x 22-11 Overhead Rope Triceps

- 4 x 11 Single Handle Curls *superset with*
- 4 x 11 Single Handle Reverse Triceps

- 4 x 11 Heavy Barbell Curls
- 4 x 11 Heavy Close Grip Benches

9 TRICEPS & BICEPS
(37 sets/ 539 reps)

- 3 x 22 Standing Alternating Dumbbell Curls *superset with*
- 3 x 11 Dumbbell Throwbacks

- 4 x 22-11 Decline Skull Crushers   *superset with*
- 3 x 22 Bench Dips

- 4 x 22-11 Overhead Rope Triceps   *superset with*
- 4 x 22-11 Low Cable Curls

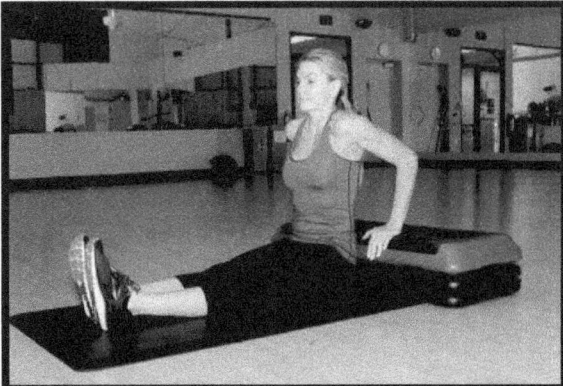

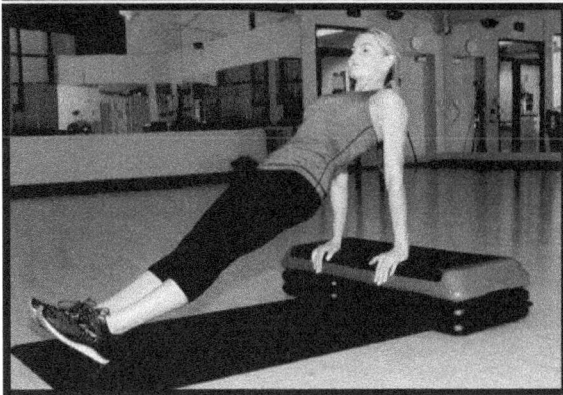

BENCH DIPS

- 4 x 11 Single Handle Curls   *superset with*
- 4 x 11 Reverse Single Handle Triceps Pulldowns

These two moves are finishing, specific movements that require great concentration for proper range of motion and attention to detail for the biceps and triceps. Do them with focused control and perfect execution.

Then move on the next *Superset.*

to

- 4 x 11 Heavy

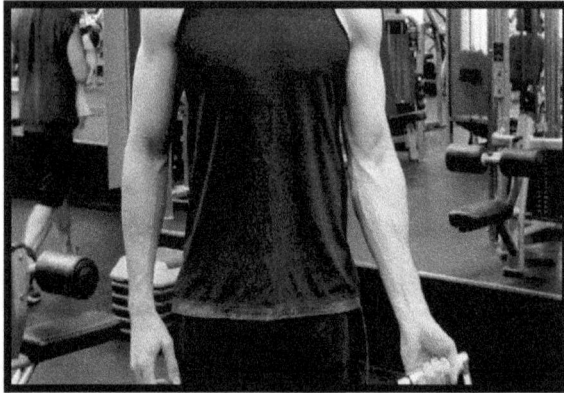

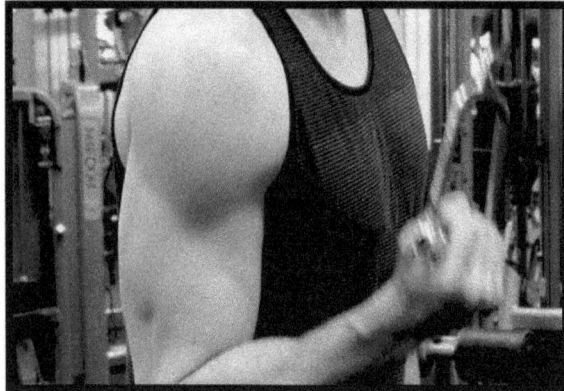

Straight Barbell Curls   *superset with*
- 4 x 11 Heavy Close-grip Benches

#10 "4 x 6" WORKOUT TRICEPS & BICEPS

(16 sets/ 528 reps)

Add weight up to 11's, dropping down to 33's
All separate sets, exercise by exercise movement.
- 33, 22, 11, 11, 22, 33 Preacher Curls
- 33, 22, 11, 11, 22, 33 Close Grip Bench Press
- 33, 22, 11, 11, 22, 33 Incline Dumbbell Curl
- 33, 22, 11, 11, 22, 33 Triceps Cable Pushdowns

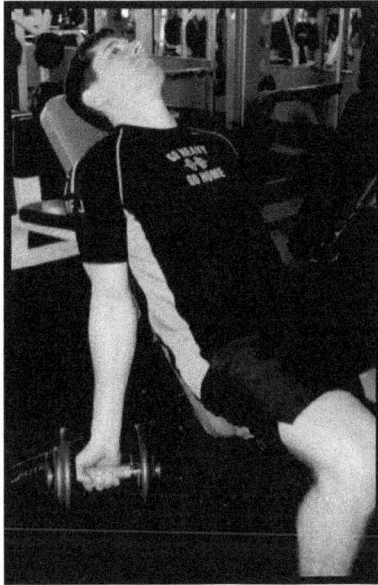

INCLINE DUMBBELL CURL

#11 BICEPS / TRICEPS/ FOREARMS
(31 sets/ 528 reps)

- 4 x 22-11 Close-grip Bench Press   *superset with*
- 4x22-11 Barbell Curls

- 4 x 22-11 Triceps Overhead Ropes   *superset with*
- 4 x 22 Alternating Dumbbell Curls

- 3 x 22 Triceps Pushdowns   *superset with*
- 3 x 22 Close-grip Bicep Cable Curls

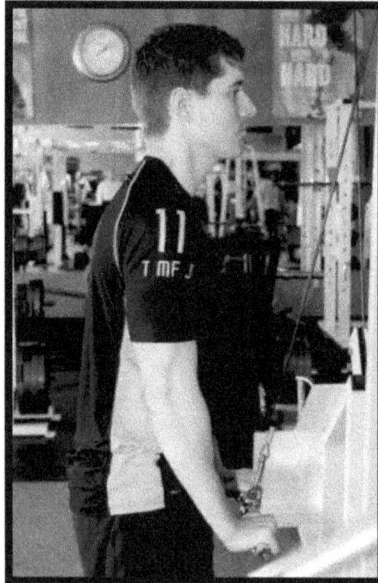

TRICEPS PUSHDOWNS

FOREARMS
Superset all three

(See Pages 48-49)

- 3 x 11 Reverse Curls – thumbs around the bar, hands just wider than shoulder width
- 3 x 22 Wrist Curls – bending the wrists downward, but not extending the fingertips
- 3 x 11 Zottman Curls – also called Hammers, keep elbows tucked at sides, back straight

All racquet sports require great forearm strength. Many instruments require great forearm strength to hold notes and sounds for long periods. Golf, hockey, baseball and any recreational sport require strength and stamina in the forearms.

BICEPS & TRICEPS -
THE MONSTER IN THE CLOSET (32 sets/ 528 reps)
Part A)- finish all these first, then B
- 4 x 22-11 Close Grip Benches
- 4 x 22-11 Triceps Pushdowns
- 4 x 22-11 Standing Barbell Curls
- *4 x 11-22 Zottman Curls Seated

Part B) – done in rapid succession - superset
- 4 x 22-11 Incline Dumbbell Curls
- 4 x 22-11 Rope Pulldowns
- 4 x 22-11 Overhead Rope Pulls
- *4 x 11-22 Close Grip Cable Curls

*Pay attention to the alternated rep schemes on these 4 movements

Each of these workouts should be done in an hour or less. The Monster is really hard to fit in, you have to have a perfect set up and again, it's best to work with a partner on as many of these as possible. It mainly helps eliminate rest time, which is crucial to the effectiveness of these Shock And Awe© workouts.

The number one goal is to perform all the reps, and not just "going through the motions." You must perform them as fully and perfectly as possible to cut the deep grooves into the muscles that bring out details and make all the connections strong. We desire "NO WEAK LINKS!" If you are only pumping the center of the muscle belly, you are strengthening the middle while the ends, the tie-ins and connections, grow weaker. So on the high-rep sets, give extra attention to range-of-motion, almost to the point of over-exaggeration.

You may have alternative names for some of these exercises (and for Me once you're through!), but if too many are foreign, or exact execution is questioned, drop me a line on the www.shockandawemuscle.com website where I'll work to explain the movements according to your questions. Stay Pumped!

And if those weren't enough for you Arm Bandits, here is another one:

BICEPS & TRICEPS
- 3 x 22 Standing Alternating Curls   *superset with*
- 3 x 11 Dumbbell Throwbacks

- 4 x 22-11 Decline Skull Crushers   *superset with*
- 3 x 22 Dips

- 4 x 22-11 Concentrations Curls
- 4 x 22-11 Overhead Rope Triceps

- 4 x 11 Single Handle Curls   *superset with*
- 4 x 11 Single Handle Reverse Triceps

- 4 x 11 Heavy Barbell Curls
- 4 x 11 Heavy Close-grip Benches

SHOCK AND AWE© BACK

Force is generated by the legs but transferred to the arms through the trunk, the core. A strong back and abs are crucial for generating and conveying this force to the extremities, as well as protecting against opposing forces from the front in contact sports.

The back is composed of hundreds of muscles which overlap each other and run in various directions, vertically, horizontally and cross-striation. Therefore, it's important to train the back with many varied grips, angles and range of motion. Exercises where you pull in a downward direction work the taper of the back, as with pull-ups and pull-downs.

The middle back and its thickness respond from movements pulled toward the body, rows in particular. Rowing movements can be done with almost any type of equipment, from a straight chinning bar, to cables, dumbbells and barbells and a number of machines specifically designed for targeting the back.

Single handle, two-hand, horizontal grip, vertical grip, palms up or down, are all different ways to stimulate the back. When designing Back training, use a combination of apparatus to allow the greatest engagement of muscles. Optimal back training involves downward pulls, pulling the body up in varied grips; pulls toward the body, single-arm movements, iso-lateral movements and both horizontal and vertical grips.

The following Shock And Awe© Back workouts will work the back from the neck to the lumbar, from the spine out toward the "wings." Since it is such a large bodypart, it is best to train it solo when working toward gaining size, since it requires much energy and much detailed attention. The short rests required in Shock And Awe© make it even more exhausting. For general training, it pairs nicely with Chest training, utilizing the push/pull dynamics of both muscle groups.

#1 BACK

- 3x 11 Pull-ups

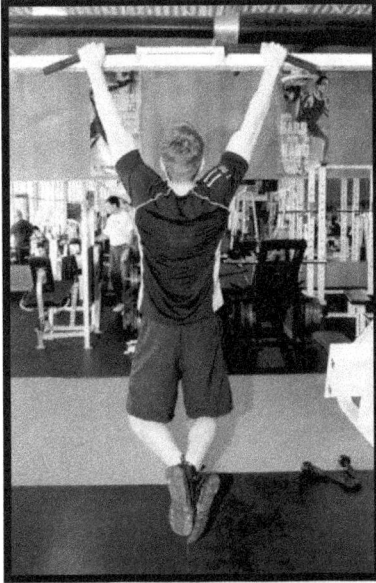

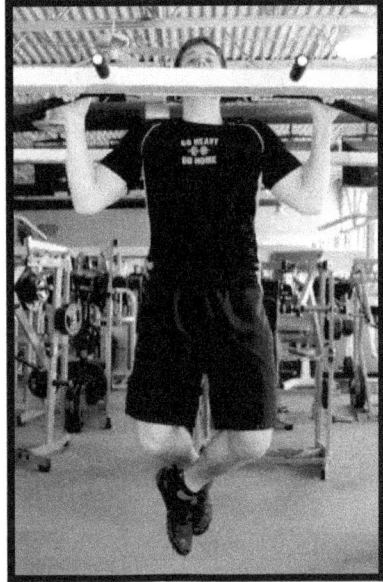

PULL-UPS

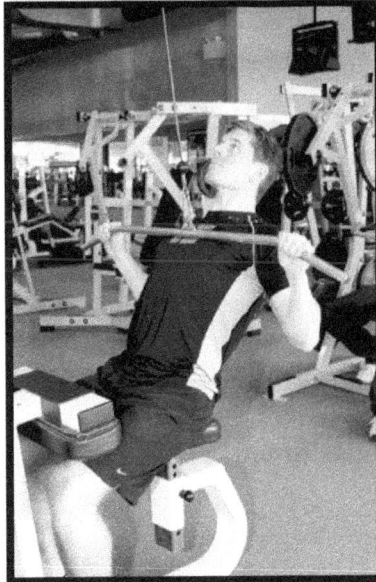

PULL-DOWNS

- 4 x 22-11 Pull-downs

You must pull these to the lower portion of the chest, at the bottom ridge, in order to fully activate the latissimus. When you pull too high, you only hit the top of the chest and do not allow the full sweep of the back muscles to develop.

- 4 x 22-11 Barbell Rows (2 w/hands on top, 2 w/hands on bottom)
- 4 x 22-11 T-bar rows

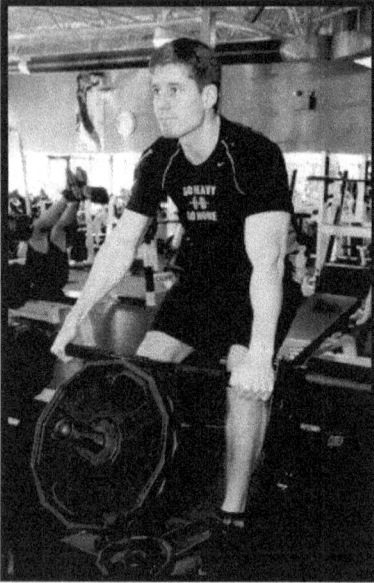

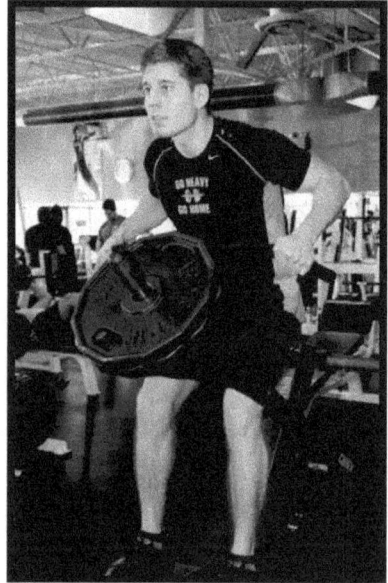

T-BAR ROWS

T-Bar Rows must be done in a semi-seated position and the form must be kept throughout. As with all back exercises, pull the elbows as high as possible without jerking through the legs or shoulders.

The position of the hands determines whether you are working on the width or the thickness; a wider grip for wider spread; narrow grip for thickness closer to the spine. The body should not follow the weight downward, you must stretch through the arms, hamstrings and lats to fully engage the back muscles.

- 4 x 11 Single Arm Rows -done heavy with a dumbbell

- 4 x 22-11 High to Low Machine Pulls – this is a Iso-lateral or comparable machine where the handles are above the head and you pull downward, squeezing at the contraction. Hold the contracted side back, lift the opposing arm, then bring fully back to hold contraction while the other arm extends.

superset with

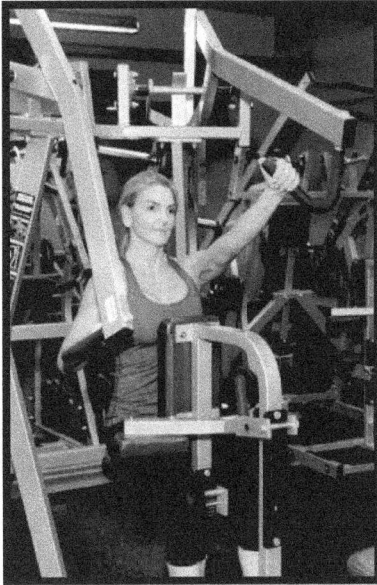

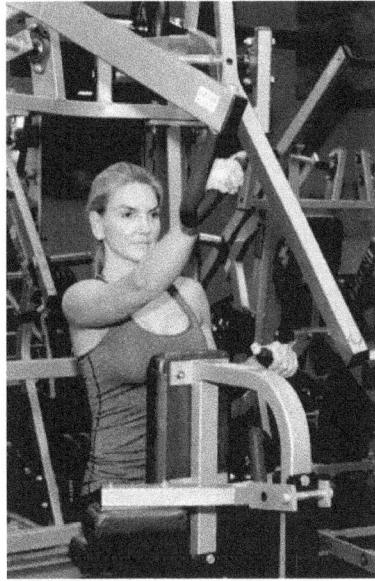

HIGH TO LOW PULLS

• 4 x 11-22 Low to High Machine Pulls – this is a Iso-lateral or comparable machine where the handles are at the waist or lower and are pulled upward toward the body and held. Hold the contracted side back, lift the opposing arm, then bring fully back to hold contraction while the other arm extends.

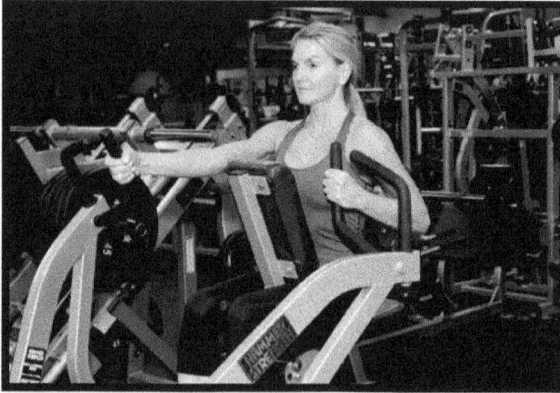

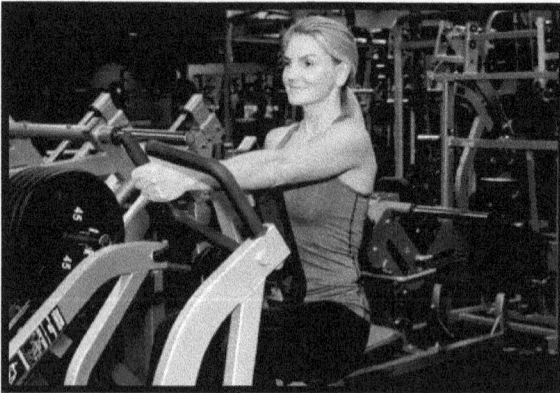

LOW TO HIGH PULLS

- 3 x 11 Hyperextensions

  superset with

- 3 x 11 Side bends each plane - left, right, center

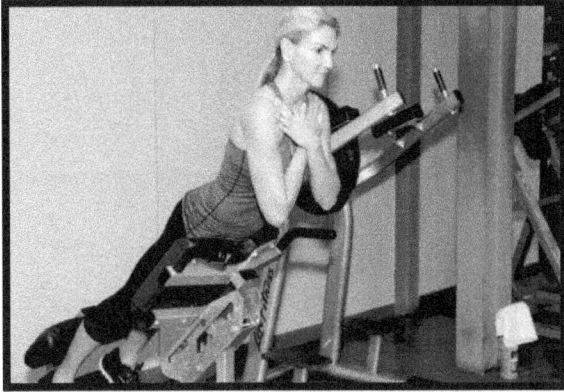

HYPEREXTENSIONS

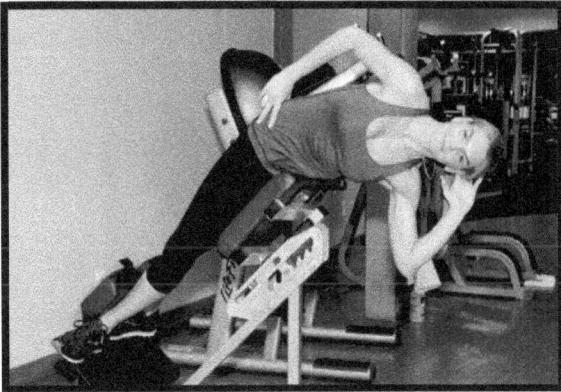

SIDE BENDS

#2 BACK

- 4 x 22-11 Barbell Rows (2 w/hands on top, 2 w/hands on bottom)
- 4 x 22-11 T-bar rows
- 3 x 11-22 High Pull to Low Machine

superset with

- 3 x 22-11 Low Pull to High Machine
- 4 x 11 Heavy Deadlifts

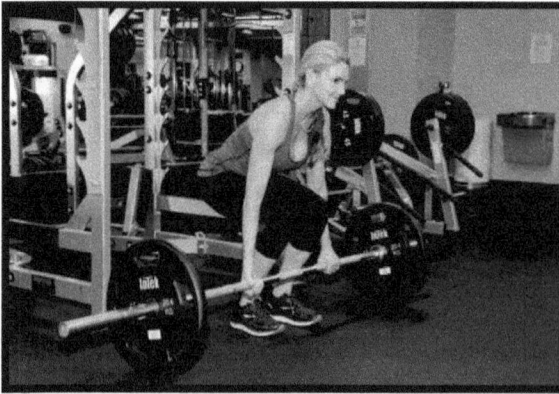

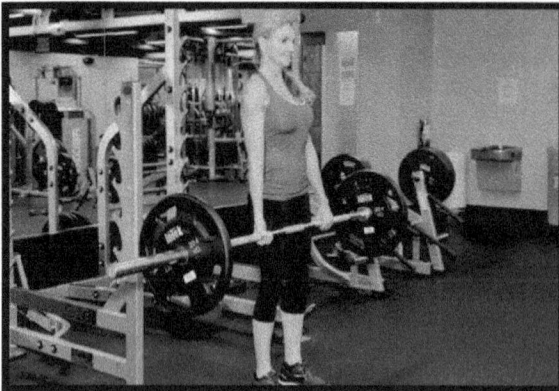

DEADLIFTS

• 3 x 11 Single Handle Cable Rows – on a Seated Pulley Row machine, the feet on the floor, back straight, pull thumb back to lowest rib and hold for a two-count.

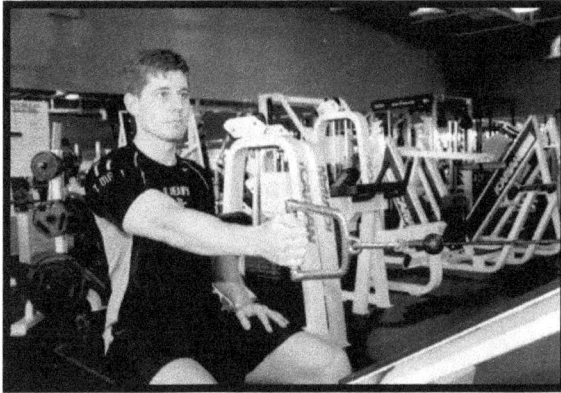

SINGLE HANDLE CABLE ROWS

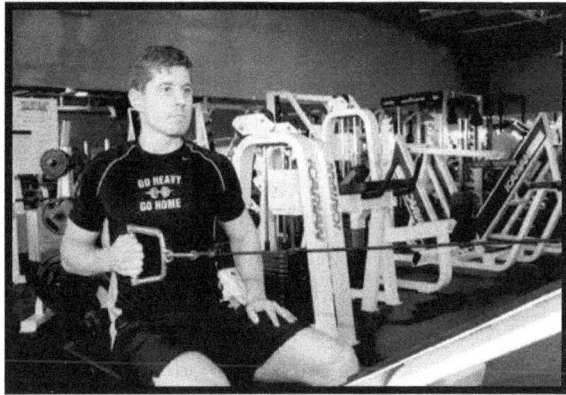

superset with

• 3 x 11 Single Handle Pulldowns – ideally, the apparatus has both vertical and horizontal pulley stations. This is the vertical plane, pulling from a high position toward the body. (Not Shown)

• 3 x 11 Rear Shoulder Machine Pulls – these are done on a reverse pec-deck machine, thumbs pointed down, chin level, ribcage high, elbows locked to full expansion.

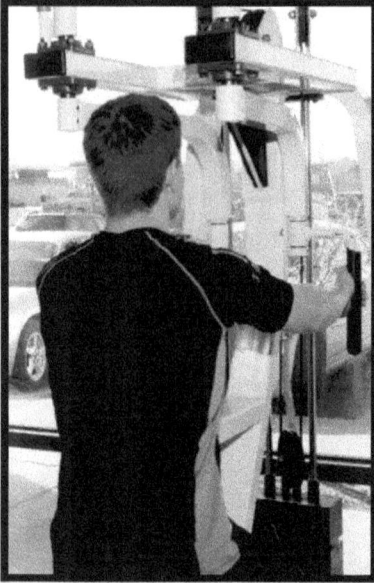

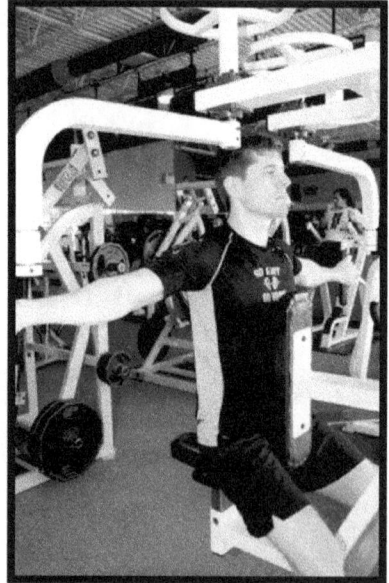

These Machine Pulls are done facing in toward a Pec Deck. You must pull the handles straight out to the sides, without pulling through the Triceps or Biceps. The purpose is to work the Rhomboid muscles between the shoulder blades by forcing the pull to come from the center of the back and lower deltoids, rather than pulling through the arms.

Use light weight and think of falling back into a backward swan dive. The arms should be straight out from the shoulders at the top of the movement, with a hold outward to feel the rhomboids engaged throughout.

- 3 x 11 Side-Bends on Swiss Ball or Hyperextension Chair – to each side, and to the center in a lower back raise down the middle; so, you do left, center, right, then next movement
superset with
- 3 x 22 Kickups (on Swiss Ball) – lay on belly with hands on floor for support, raise both legs from the lumbar of the back, rather than with momentum from the heels.

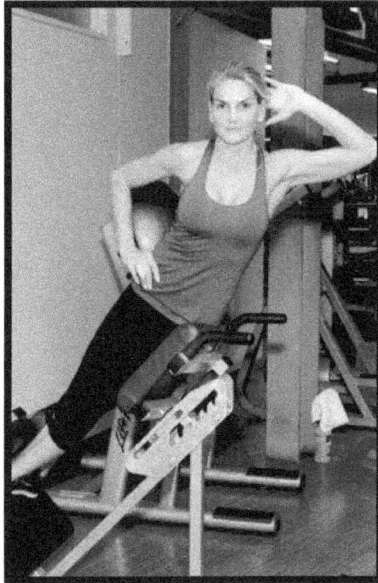

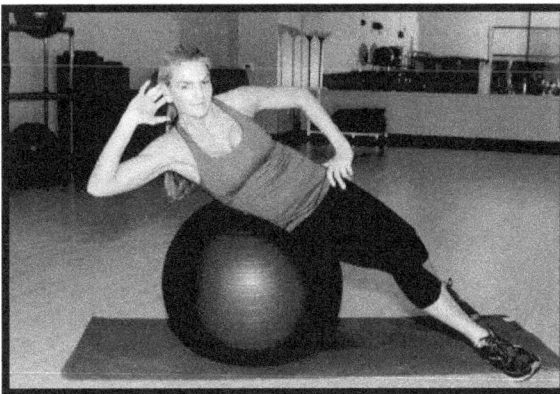

#3 BACK

- 3 x 11 Pull-ups on Graviton – this is the weight-assisted pull-up machine
- 4 x 22-11 Seated Pulley Rows –legs straight, ribcage high, pull fully back and reach fully forward through the shoulders rather than bending at the waist to reach
- 4 x 22-11 Pull-downs

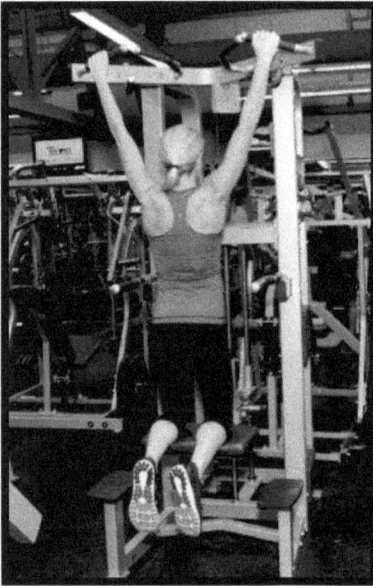

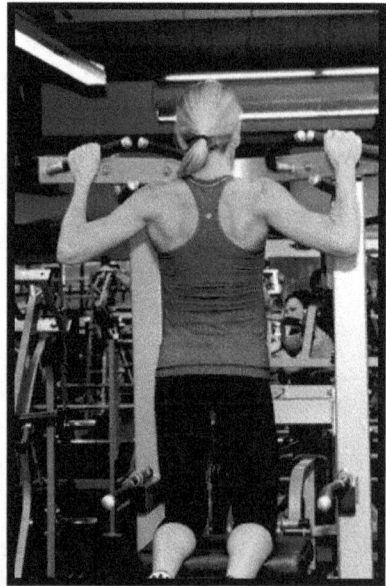

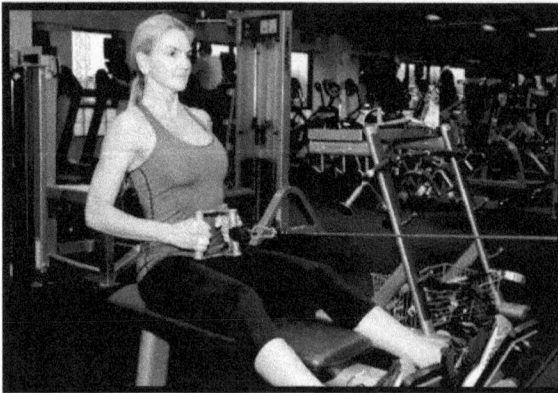

- 4 x 11 T-Bar Rows (go heavy on these with all you have left) – legs bent, head high
- 3 x 22 Side Bends on hyperextension machine or ball
- 3 x 22 Good Mornings - with straight bar across neck, bend at waist, keep legs straight.
- 3 x 22 Flat Back Crunches – lay on ground, knees bent, feet flat, elbows wide and relaxed.

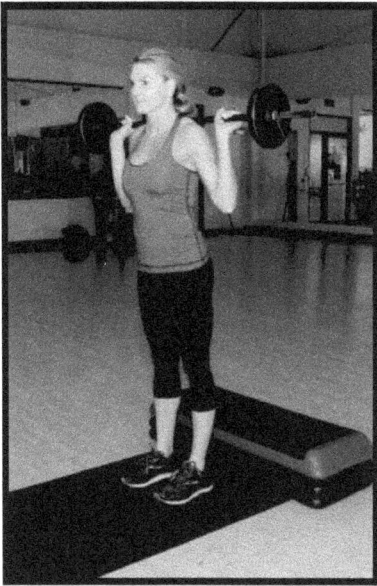

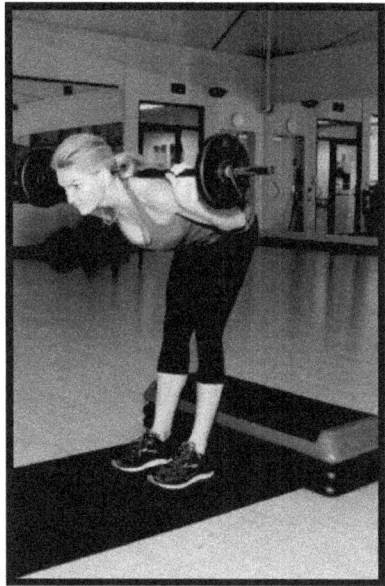

GOOD MORNINGS

#4 Trapezius/Upper Back Workout

• 3 x 11 Pull-ups Behind Neck

superset with

• 3 x 22 Pull-downs Behind Neck

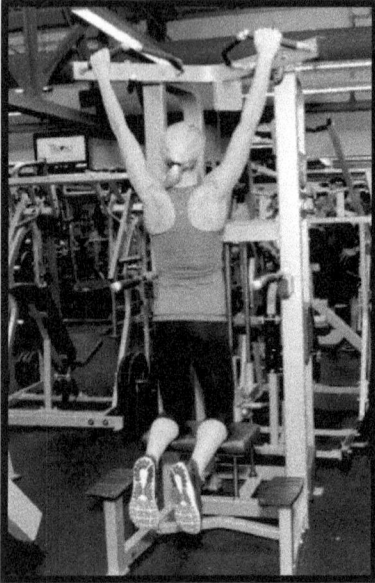 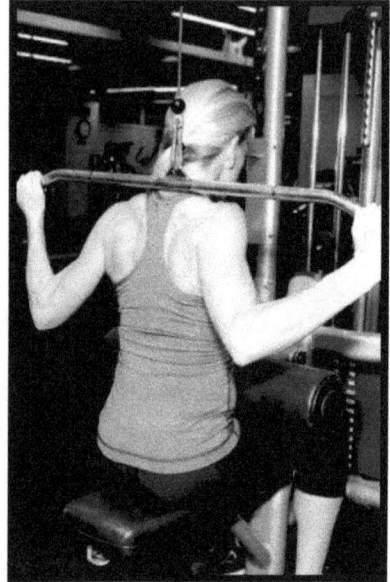

PULL UPS   *PULL DOWNS*

- 4 x 22-11 Rear Shrugs on Smith Machine – bar is behind butt, fingers pointing backward, raise shoulders to ears.

  superset with

- 4 x 11-22 Front Shrugs on Smith Machine – bar in front of thighs, fingers face forward, raise shoulders to ears.

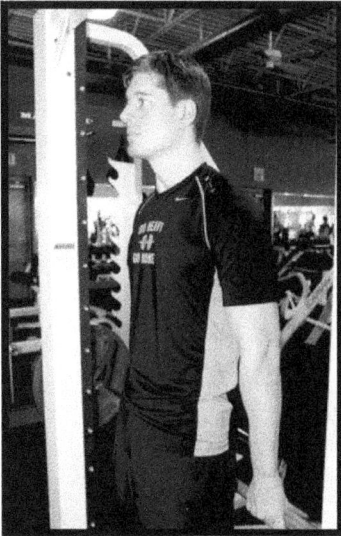 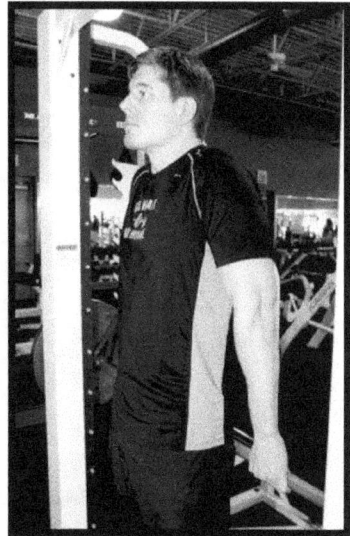

R
E
A
R

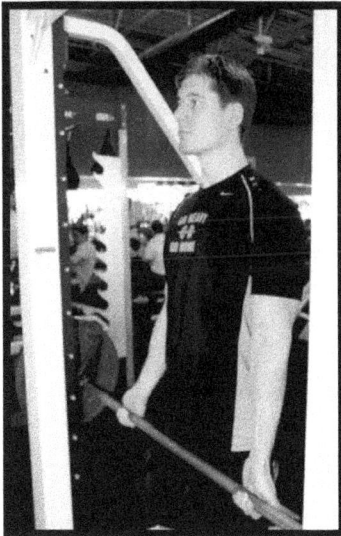 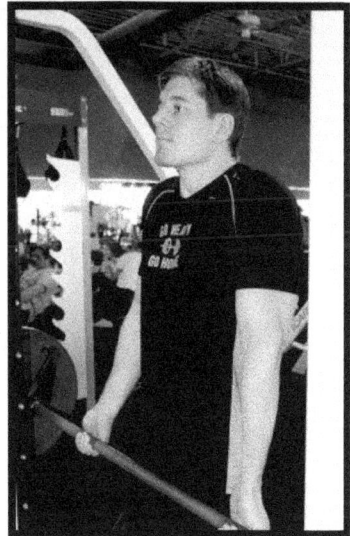

F
R
O
N
T

- 4 x 11 Dumbbell Hangs – heavy dumbbells, hands at sides, slight up and down moves. These are similar to Shrugs (shown above) but with dumbbells, the stress goes to the outer portion of the trapezius group.

superset with

- 4 x 11 Seated Pulley Row To Neck – with short handle, keep elbows high and parallel to floor, pull bar slowly and fully to chin with back straight and weight light. Perfect form.

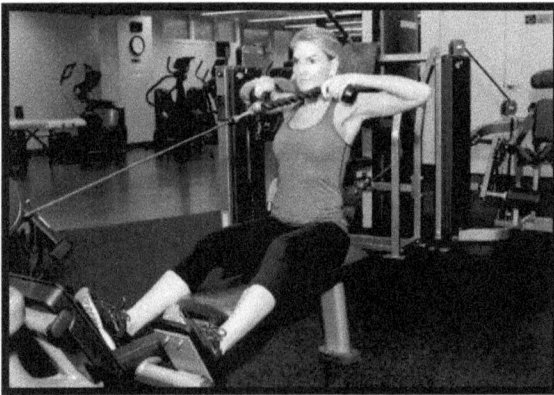

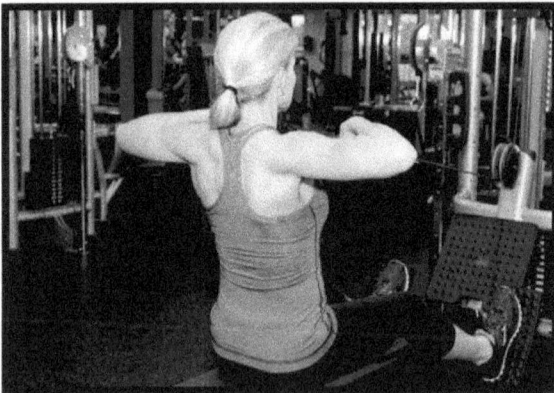

SEATED PULLEY ROW TO NECK

#5 RHOMBOID SPECIFIC BACK WORKOUT

The rhomboids, a diamond-shaped cluster located in the center of the back between the shoulder-blades, are the posture muscles. The larger muscles of the back take the brunt of the workload off these smaller muscles. The rhomboids require great concentration to isolate and activate. Isometric exercises are initially effective to stress them, but once you can feel direct work through them, you can add weight and strength. These are vital in racket and any swing sports, or rowing and climbing activities. You also cannot help standing up straighter.

- 3 x 22 Rhomboid Rows – Hold dumbbells at sides, sit upright, head back, pull shoulder blades together. superset with
- 3 x 11 Dumbbell Horizontal Pulls – standing, grasp light dumbbells so thumbs point up. Pull arms to sides while chin stays high and elbows remain locked.   *superset with*

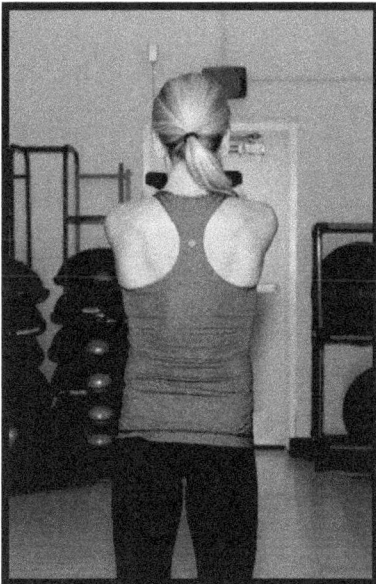

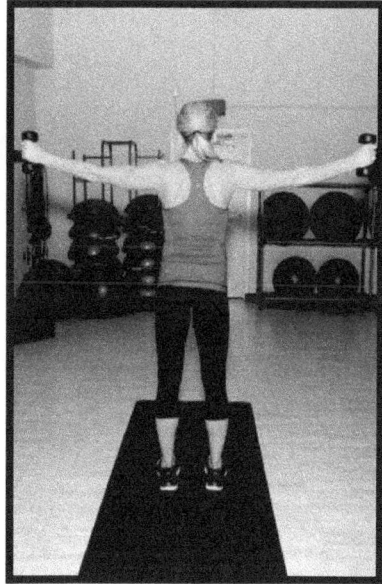

- 3 x 22 Olympic Bar Shoulder Lifts – laying flat on a bench, hold a barbell at arms length with elbows locked, press outward using just the middle back. Add weight as necessary.

superset with

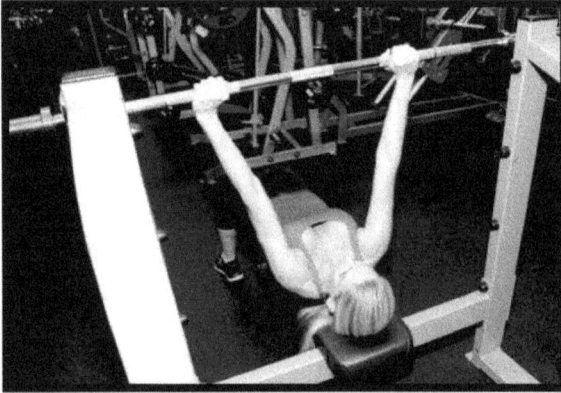

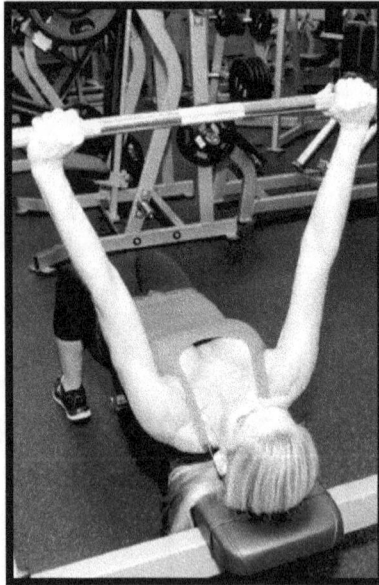

SHOULDER LIFTS

- 3 x 11 Straight Bar Drops – standing, grasp a barbell outside shoulder width, raise to eye level, then extremely slowly, let descend to thighs; raise and resume repetitions.

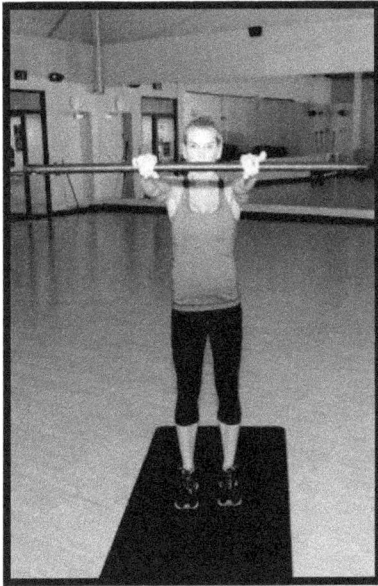

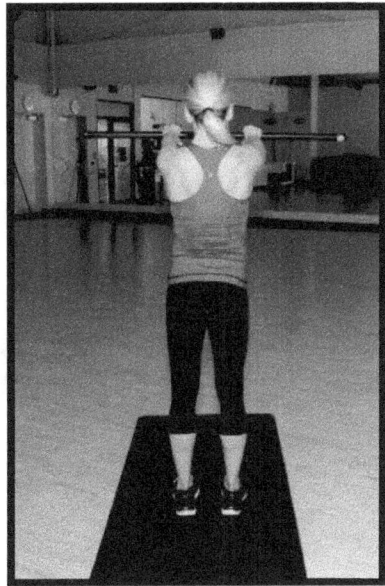

STRAIGHT BAR DROPS

In order to fully feel this movement, concentrate on the spine in relation to where the bar drops in front of you. As it falls, you should feel the corresponding tightness down the spine, along the ridge of muscles the length of your back. Use enough weight to feel this, but not too much to have to throw the weight into position. It should be a slow raise and a slower drop.

SHOCK AND AWE - *BICEPS*

These are great workouts that stand on their own, but can be teamed with other bodyparts, like Triceps or Back or Chest or Legs, depending on your priorities.

#1 BICEPS

• 4 x 22-11 Barbell Curls w/Straight Bar – thumbs tucked in "Monkey Grip" under bar.

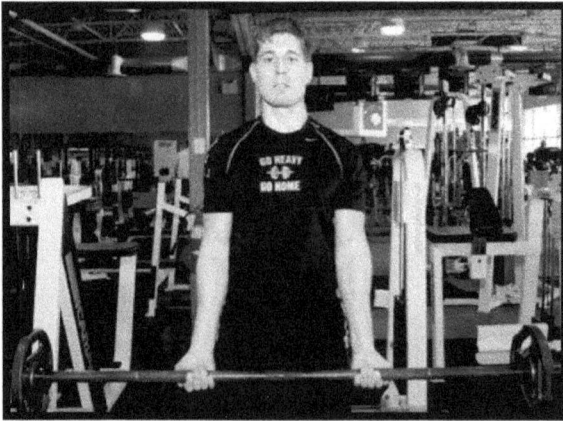

STANDING BARBELL CURL

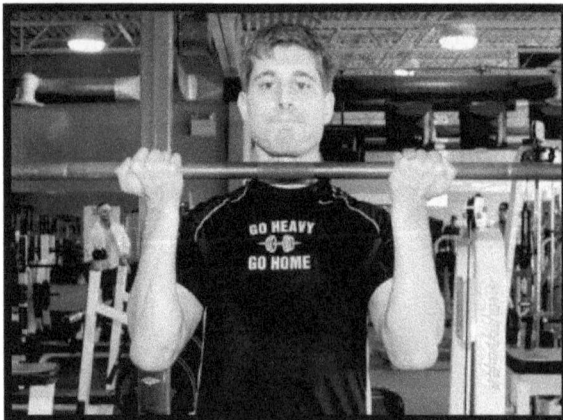

- 4 x 22-11 45° Incline Dumbbell Curls - with head to bench, full extension of arms straight down, full curl at top.

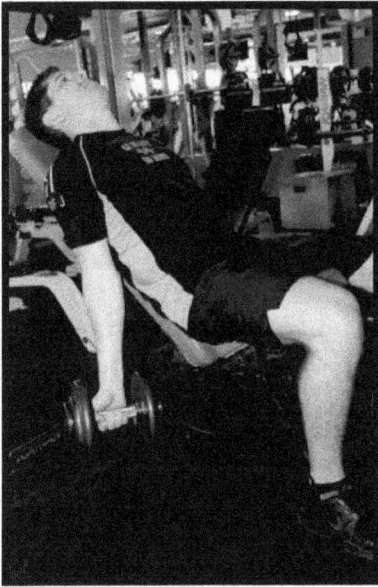

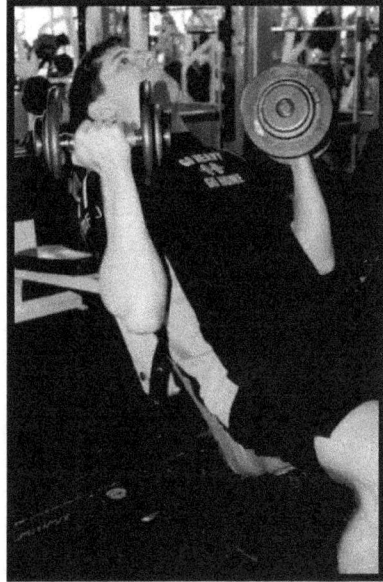

45° INCLINE DUMBBELL CURLS

45° INCLINE DUMBBELL CURLS are fantastic for lower, outer Biceps development because the stretch involved forces the outer Biceps to stay stable, while the center works hard to keep each repetition in a uniform groove.

You will get more fullness out of this movement than anything else but the Barbell Curl. With the head back, you will feel the stress across the Biceps muscles from the elbow insertion to the top at its shoulder insertion.

- 3 x 22 Seated Pulley Curls – short handle on pulley row machine, elbows at sides, reach forward, keeping elbows low.

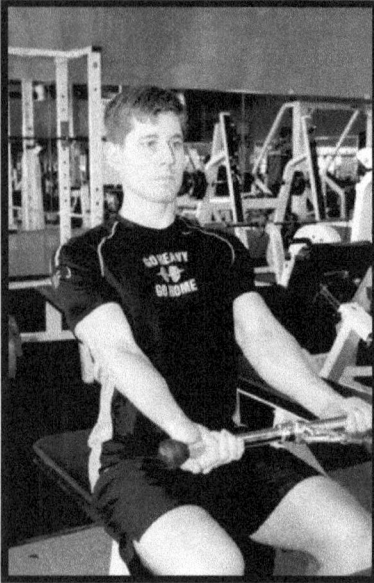

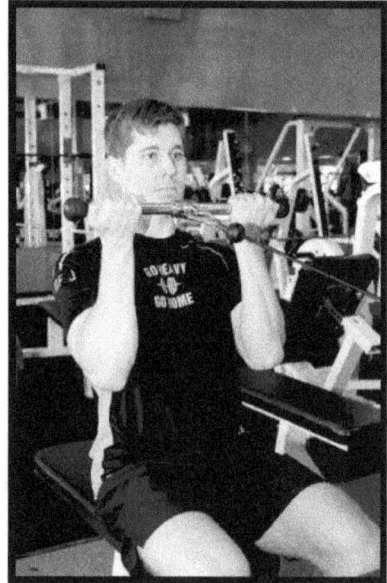

Seated Pulley Curls are one of the best exercises for putting a "peak" on the biceps. They must be done strictly, without any sway from the back, or extra pull through the upper body to move the weight up to the chin. If you force your hands away from the body at the top of the movement, the stress is on the lower outer portion of the Biceps; if you curl your fingers back toward the body at the top, more stress goes to pushing the peak upward, as they should be done.

#2 BICEPS

- 4 x 22-11 Standing Barbell Curls
- 4 x 11 Straight Bar Standing Preacher Curls - Heavy

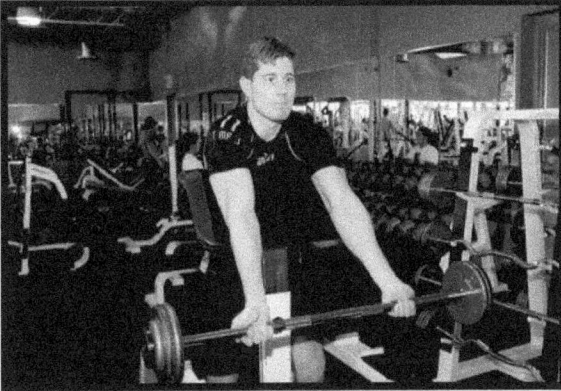

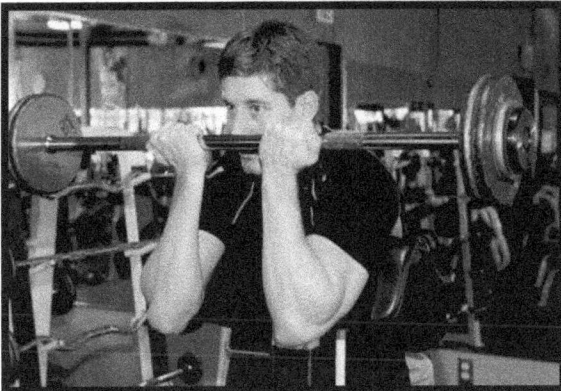

STANDING PREACHER CURLS

• 3 x 11 each Dumbbell Standing Preacher Curls – hip against the bench, arm straight.

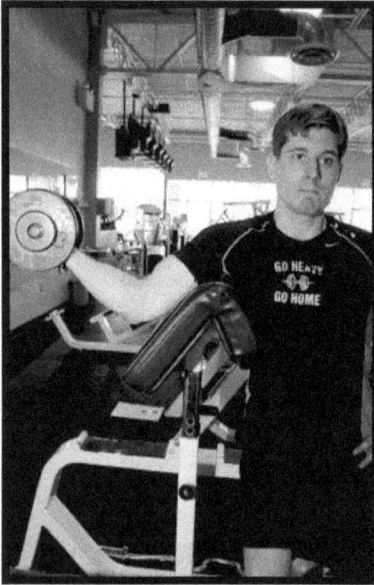

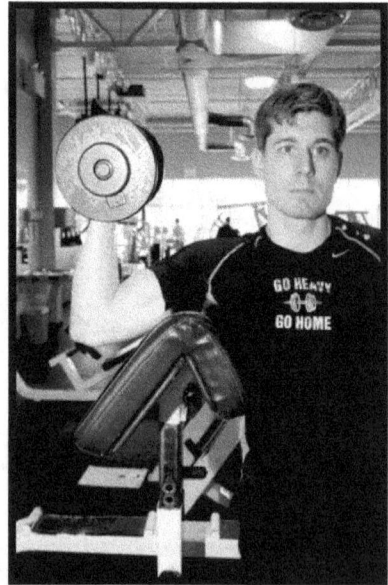

DUMBBELL STANDING PREACHER CURLS

It is good to do both the Standing Dumbbell Preacher and the Standing Barbell Preacher on any Biceps workout. You can do one each day, or both on the same day. You will notice a greater stress near the elbow on a Dumbbell Curl, and a greater stress on the top peak of the Biceps with a Barbell Curl. Both have a great gravitational pull on the arms, but it's important to keep the hips and shoulders perpendicular to the bench on the Dumbbell version; and the back straight and chest high on the Barbell version, so as to avoid leaning over the bench and rounding the shoulders forward.

#3 BICEPS

- 4 x 22 -11 Barbell Curls
- 11, 11, 11, 33 Barbell Preacher Curls – add weight first 3 sets, then drop incrementally last set

- 4 x 22 Alternating Dumbbell Curls – with twist at top over biceps head and then   superset with
- 4 x 11 Throwbacks – elbows stay stationary on hips, curl toward the outside at the biceps-brachialas tie in to target the lower-outer biceps.

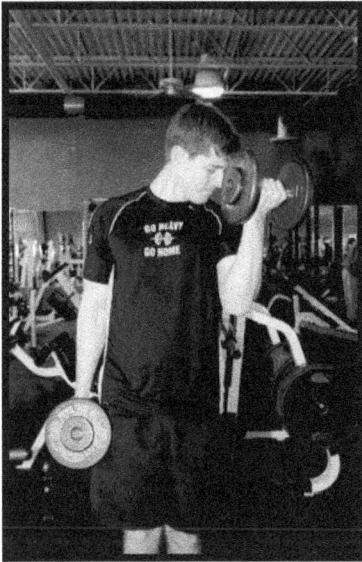

ALTERNATING CURLS

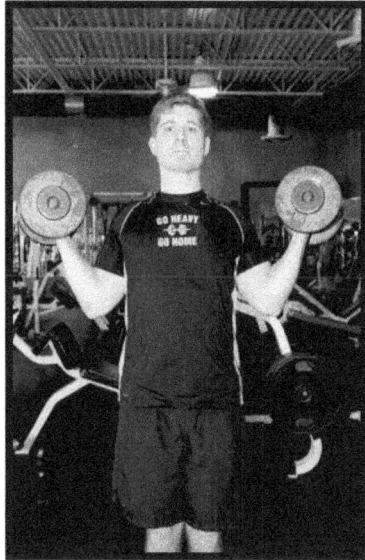

DUMBBELL THROWBACKS

#4 BICEPS

- 4 x 22-11 Straight Bar Curls
- 4 x 22-11 45° Incline Dumbbell Curls
- 4 x 11 each Single Handle Preacher Curls
- 4 x 22-11 Seated Barbell Preacher Curls

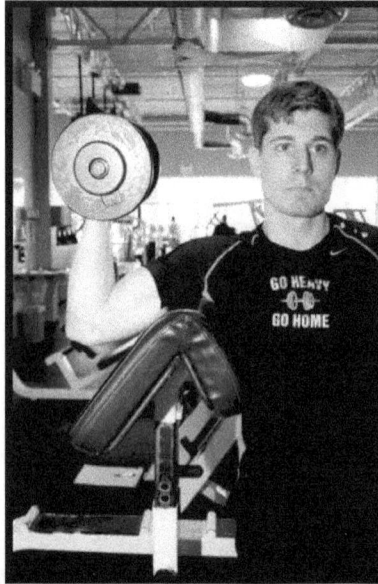

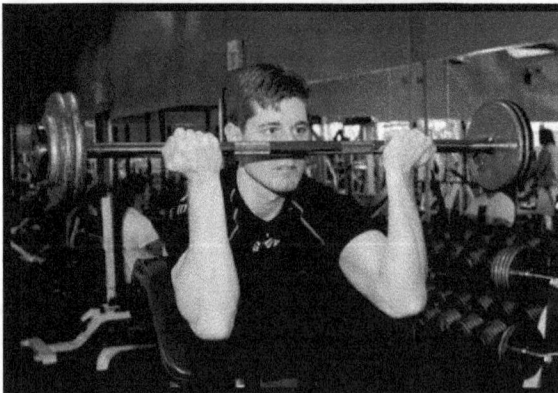

SEATED BARBELL PREACHER CURLS

#5 BICEPS

- 4 x 22-11 Standing Barbell Curls
- 4 x 22-11 Incline Dumbbell Curls
- 3 x 22 Seated Pulley Curls

#6 BICEPS

- 3x 22 Standing Alternate Dumbbell Curls *superset with*
- 3 x 22 Preacher Straight Bar Curls *superset with*
- 3 x 11 Heavy E-Z Bar Curls
- 4 x 22-11 Barbell Curls

- 3 x 22 Dumbbell Incline Curls *superset with*
- 3 x 11 Dumbbell Concentration Curls – done standing with arm perpendicular to floor

CONCENTRATION CURLS

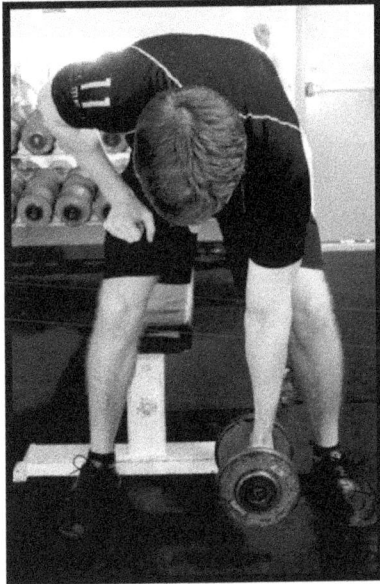

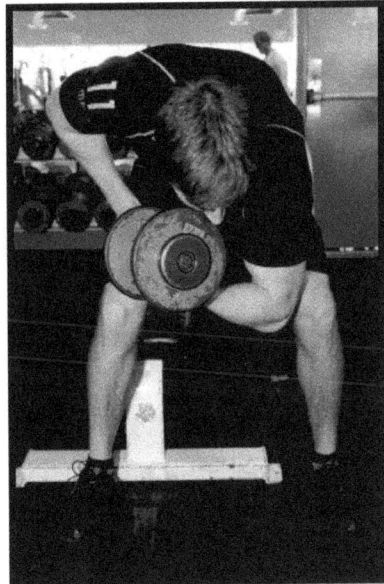

81

#7 BICEPS

- 4 x 22 Standing Alternating Curls
  superset with
- 4 x 22-11 Throwback Curls

- 4 x 11 each Single Handle Curls
- 4 x 11 Heavy Barbell Curls
- 3 x 22 Seated Close -grip Cable Curls

#8 BICEPS

- 3 x 22 Standing Alternating Dumbbell Curls
  superset with
- 3 x 11 Dumbbell Throwbacks

- 4 x 22-11 Low Cable Curls
- 4 x 11 Single Handle Curls
- 4 x 11 Heavy Straight Barbell Curls

#9 BICEPS

- 33, 22, 11, 11, 22, 33 Preacher Curls – adding weight up to 11's, dropping weight down to 33's
- 33, 22, 11, 11, 22, 33 Incline Dumbbell Curl

#10 BICEPS

- 4 x 22-11 Barbell Curls
- 4 x 22 Alternating Dumbbell Curls
- 3 x 22 Close Grip Cable Curls

#11 BICEPS SUPERSET

- 4 x 22-11 Standing Barbell Curls   superset with
- 4 x 11-22 Zottman Curls Seated   superset with
- 4 x 22-11 Incline Dumbbell Curls

SHOCK AND AWE© *CHEST*

The key to making a well-defined, muscular chest is to hit it from many angles. You are a sculptor and must give it depth and aesthetic appeal from every angle. Even a small chest looks good if it's defined and well-developed.

You do this by changing the hand positions, from knuckles facing away, as in a bench press; to knuckles facing each other, as in a dumbbell press. You change the angle of the bench, higher up toward vertical for more development toward the collarbone; to decline, for hitting the lower edges of the chest. Essentially, where the bar hits, is where it's working. If you hit the center of the chest across the nipples, you work it fully, at its broadest spectrum.

If you hit near the neck, you work the upper chest, the area seen when your shirt is open. Lower, toward the bottom edge of the pectorals, you are building the lower edge. When you stretch the elbows low along the ribcage, as in a dip or dumbbell press, you are isolating the outer edges which give the chest its definition in the side view.

#1 CHEST

- 2 x 22-11 Bent-over Cable Flyes
- 2 x 22-11 70° Standing Cable Flyes
- 4 x 22-11 Bench Press, or
- 4 x 22-11 Incline Bench Press, or
- 4 x 22-11 Decline Bench Press
- 3 x 11 Pullovers

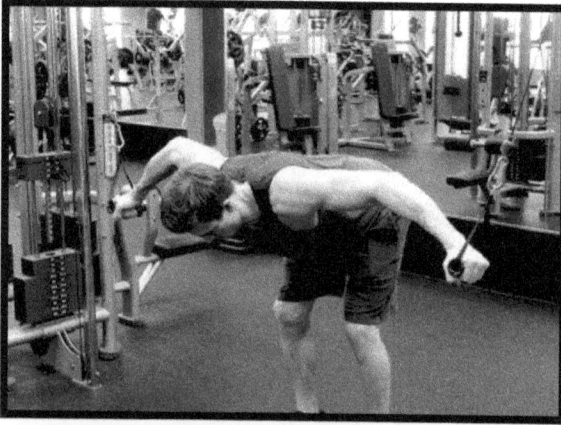

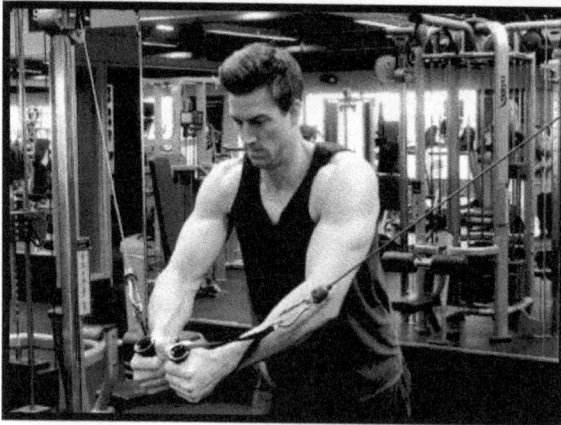

CABLE FLYES - BENT OVER & 70° STANDING

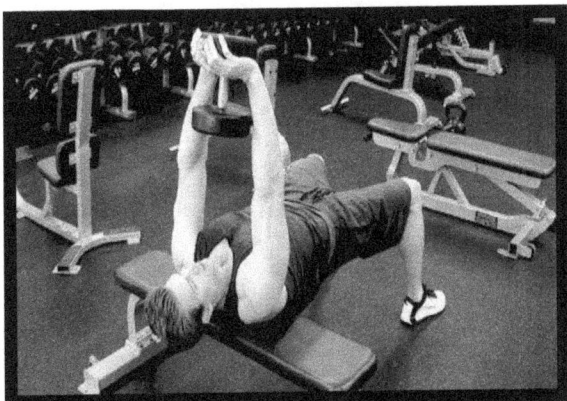

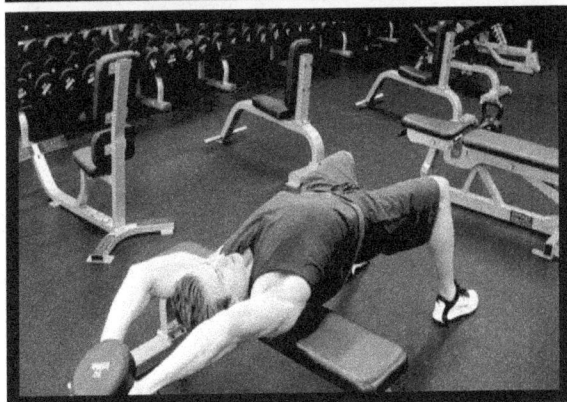

PULLOVERS

Take a deep breath on the descending aspect of this movement, hold at the top, exhale forcefully as you return it over your face. Keep the elbows locked and reach back, rather than down toward the floor. The hips should be slightly lower than the shoulders to enable the ribcage to fully expand.

#2 CHEST (Outer Edges Focus)

- 3 x 11 Dips

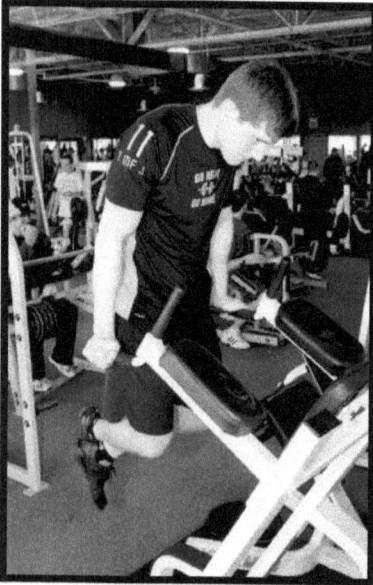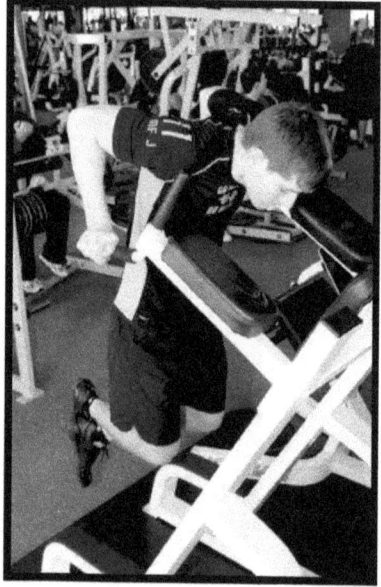

DIPS

- 2 x 22-11 Bent-over Cable Flyes
- 2 x 22-11 70° Standing Cable Flyes

You make your chest big by giving it depth. It does not matter how much weight you can lift, it matters how equally proportionate and defined the pectoral muscles develop. The best and only way to acquire this, is to go through the full range of motion on all movements. The Chest does not require tons of weight to grow; it requires tons of attention and focus on where the movement is affecting the musculature. You can focus on the lower, outer or upper regions of the Chest; but a balanced approach is best; because you'll only spend undo amounts of time correcting the differences.

- 2 x 22-11 Low To High Cable Flyes – from low position on pulleys, reach from behind to full extension in front of face, coming up in a smooth, upward arc rather than a line. Let the knuckles face upward throughout the movement.

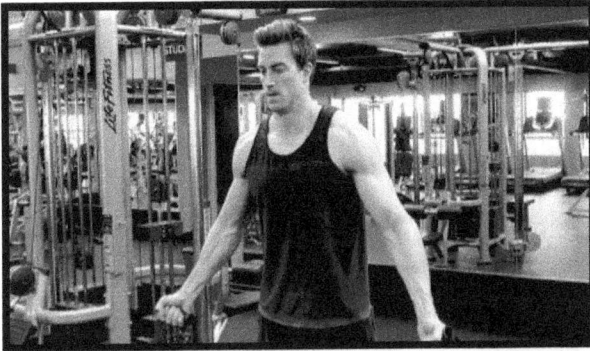

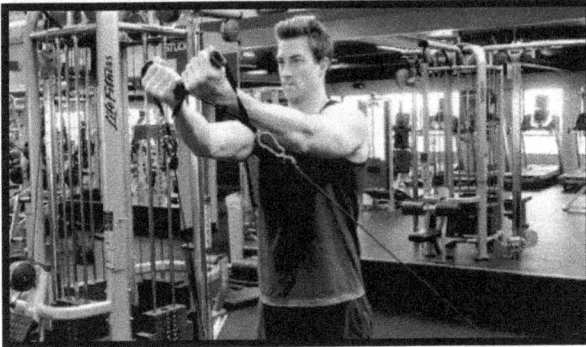

LOW TO HIGH CABLE FLYES

• 3 x 20 each side Twin T Towers - on an incline bench, hold two dumbbells over the center of chest, arms extended, always pushing both to center over chest so the tension can be felt along the collarbones. Do 5 left, 5 right, 5 left, 5 right; 4 rounds for total of 20 per side.

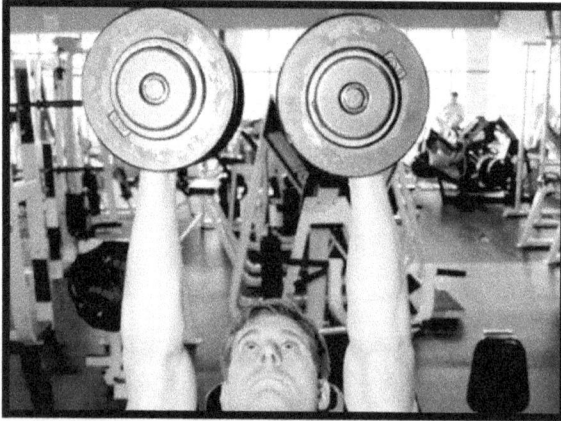

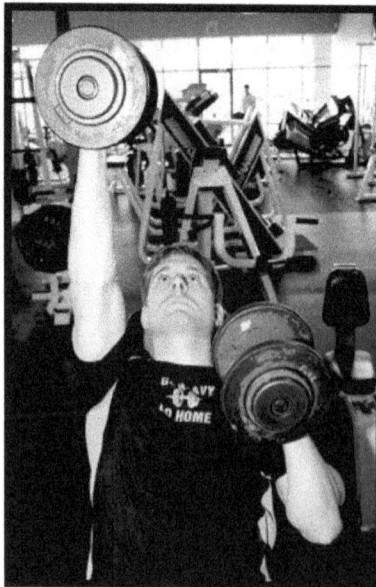

TWIN T TOWERS

- 4 x 11 Decline Bench Press - heavy
- 4 x 11 Flat Bench Press - strict and stopping at the top, slow and very concentrated

- 4 x 22-11 Peck Deck - hold strict form on the higher reps, with the top knuckles coming together on a consistent tempo with the elbows held high; and squeeze on the lower, toward the small fingers on the sets of 11, to accentuate the lower edges.

#3 CHEST

- 3x11 Dips
- 4x11 Flat Bench With Barbell – done on a regular bench, not a Smith
- 4x11 Incline Bench with Dumbbells - knuckles facing ribcage
- 3x22 Decline Dumbbell Flyes - not too heavy, watch the shoulders

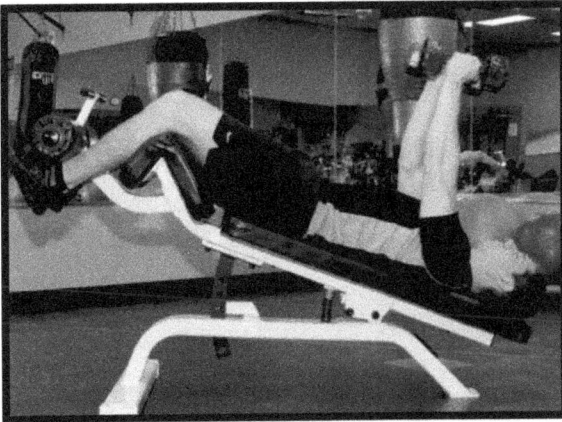

DECLINE DUMBBELLS FLYES

#4 CHEST

- 4 x 22-11 Flat Bench Press
- 4 x 22-11 Decline Bench press
- 3 x 20 each side Twin T Towers - on an incline bench, hold two dumbbells over the center of chest, arms extended, always pushing both to center over chest so the tension can be felt along the collarbones. Do 5 left, 5 right, 5 left, 5 right for total of 20 per side.

#5 CHEST

- 4 x 22-11 Pec Deck - hold strict form on the higher reps and squeeze on the lower
- 4 x 22-11 Flat Bench
- 3 x 22 Incline Dumbbell Press – knuckles to ribcage

3 x 11 Cable Flyes   *superset with*
3 x 11 Dips

3 x 11 Decline Flyes   *superset with*
3 x 11 Decline Pushups

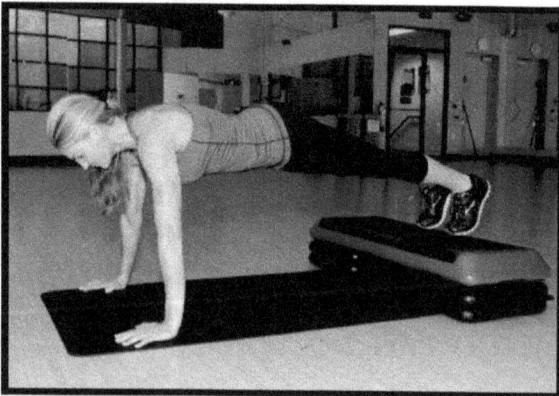

DECLINE PUSHUPS

6 CHEST

- 3 x 11 Dips
- 4 x 22-11 Smith-machine bench press
- 4 x 11 Flat Bench Dumbbell Press – with squeeze at top
- 4 x 22-11 Dumbbell Flyes
- 3 x 20 each side Twin T Towers
- 4 x 22-11 Cable Crossover Flyes – two positions, all the way down, and 70°

7 CHEST

- 3 x 11 Dips
- 4 x 22-11 Decline Bench Press – bar should hit across lower ridge of pectorals
- 3 x 20 per side Twin T Towers
- 4 x 22-11 Flat Bench Press- with narrow grip and 2-second squeeze at top
- 4 x 22-11 Pec Deck Flyes – hold strict form on the higher reps and squeeze on the lower

#8 CHEST

- 4x 22-11 Flat Bench Press
- 4x 22-11 Incline Dumbbell Presses
- 3x22 Cable Crossovers

#9 CHEST

- 3 x 22 Cable Crossovers – 3 positions, all the way down; up at 70°; standing straight up
- 4 x 22-11 Incline Bench Press – bring bar right to collarbone, very strictly
- 4 x 22-11 Flat Bench Dumbbell Flyes – keep stationary arc in arms, dropping low to sides

#10 CHEST

- 2 x 22-11 Bent-over Cable Flyes
- 2 x 22-11 70° Upright Cable Flyes
- 4 x 22-11 Decline Bench Press
- 4 x 22-11 Incline Bench Press
- 4 x 11 Pullovers
- 2 x 22-11 Low Cable Flyes - from low position to face height
- 4 x 11 Flat Bench Press - strict and stop to squeeze at the top

#11 CHEST

- 3 x 11 Dips
- 2 x 22-11 Bent-over Cable Flyes
- 2 x 22-11 70° Upright Cable Flyes
- 3 x 20 each side Twin T Towers
- 4 x 11 Decline Flyes
- 4 x 22-11 Pec Deck

#12 CHEST

- 4 x 22-11 Peck Dec
- 4 x 22-11 Flat Bench with Freeweight
- 4 x 20 each side Twin T Towers

3 x 11 Low Cable Flyes   *superset with*
3 x 11 Dips

3 x 11 Decline Flyes   *superset with*
3 x 11 Perfect Pushups

SHOCK AND AWE SUPERSETS - *CHEST & BACK*

Keep in mind that these are two of the largest muscle groups. They require enormous energy when training either one of them solo, so when you do these supersets, you better be well-versed in the movements and the higher repetitions.

The beauty of the Shock And Awe System is that it eases you into the movements with the light, high-rep warm-ups, and then suddenly nails you on the 3rd and 4th sets when the fatigue just begins to set in, you're using all your energy to push it up!

That's why it is so vitally important to keep the form on all your movements instead of rushing to get to the end of the repetitions. Cutting these deep, uniform grooves over the muscles, tie-ins and connections gives ultimate delineation of muscle group to muscle group, across all trained bodyparts. This is where the difference is between the person who says they "go to the gym" regularly, and you'd never know it by looking at them; and the ones who train with the great attention to detail that Shock And Awe System enforces. These elicit the "nice arms...legs...abs..." comments.

The individual Chest and Back workouts follow these supersets, and it may be best to start with them in their own superset fashion to get your body used to the full saturation of blood in the muscle belly's. You escalate to the point where you can hardly move the muscles you're training and you realize you're only halfway through the workout. This is the way you should be training all the time.

The other thing reported with the people I've trained, is that most have a noticeably greater strength in the chest or the back, and that difference should be addressed in these superset combinations. Always train the weaker, trailing bodypart first, when attention and energy are optimal. Always reach for balance in strength as well as symmetry, but especially in regard to the front and the back of body oppositions.

93

#1 CHEST/ BACK

- 2 x 11 Pull-ups – these can be done with a Graviton machine if necessary.   *superset with*
- 2 x 11 Dips

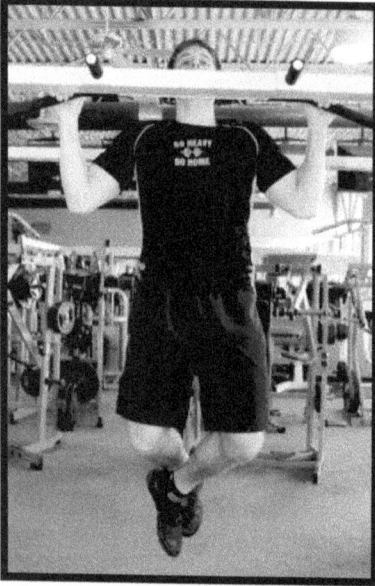

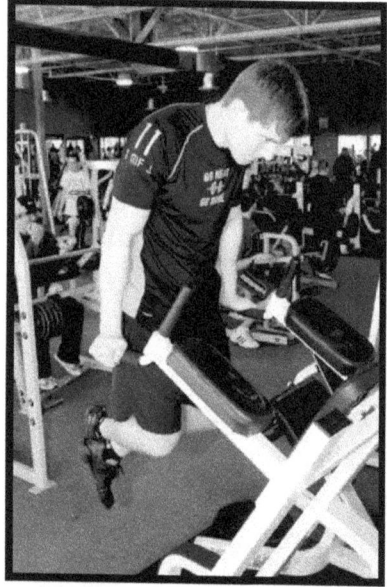

Pull-Ups are one of the best Back movements. They require strength, flexibility, and a great amount of discipline, with only a chinning bar for equipment.

Dips are one of the best exercises for the sides of the Chest. They build the outer ridge of definition that outlines the pectoral muscles and shape the chest without any extra weight required. To add weight compromises detail and puts undue stress on the shoulders.

- 4 x 22-11 Decline Bench Press – bar should hit across lower ridge of pectorals. *superset with*

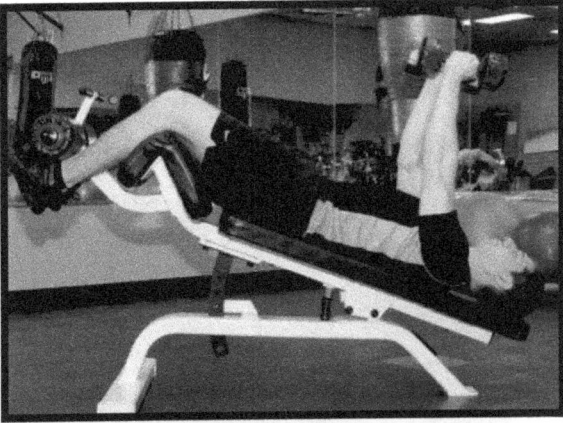

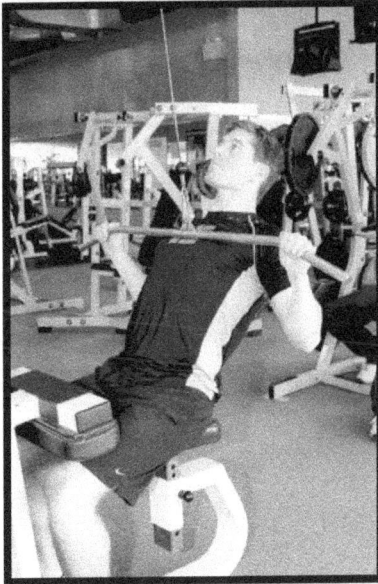

LAT PULLDOWNS

- 4 x 22-11 Lat Pulldowns to Front – lean slightly back and pull below the sternum
- 3 x 20 per side Twin T Towers – on an incline bench, hold two dumbbells over the center of chest, arms extended, always pushing both to center over chest so the tension can be felt along the collarbones.
- Do 5 left, 5 right, 5 left, 5 right for 20 repetitions each side

superset with

- 3 x 22 per side Single Dumbbell Rows

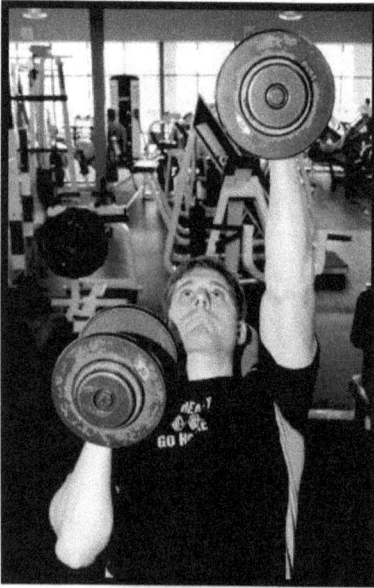 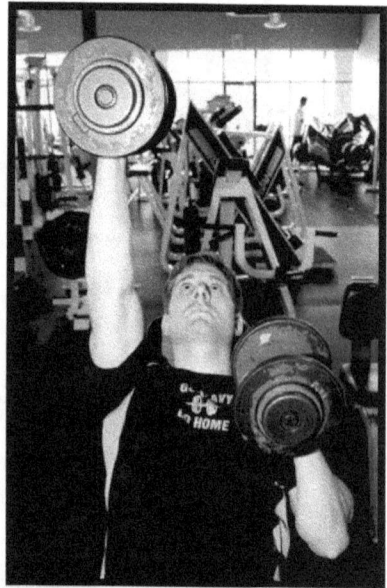

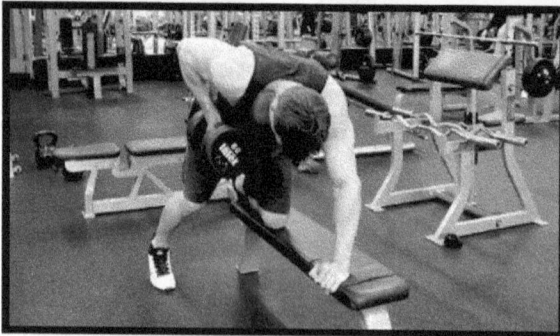

- 4 x 11 Flat Bench Press- with narrow grip and 2-second squeeze at top   *superset with*
- 4 x 11 Single Seated Pulley Rows- with squeeze contraction at pullback position.

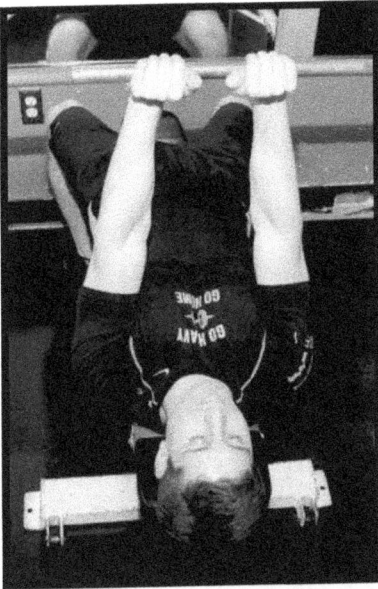

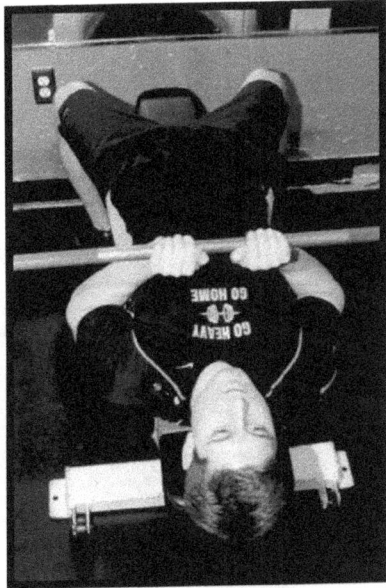

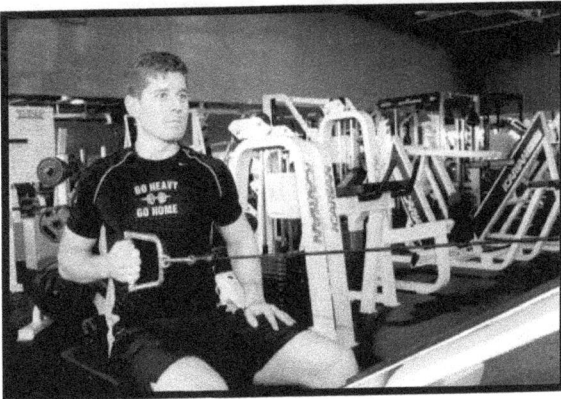

SINGLE CABLE PULLEY ROWS

- 4 x 22-11 Pec Deck Flyes – hold strict form on the higher reps and squeeze on the lower   *superset with*
- 4 x 11-22 Rhomboid Pulls to Neck- on seated pulley cable machine (see Back)

N   o

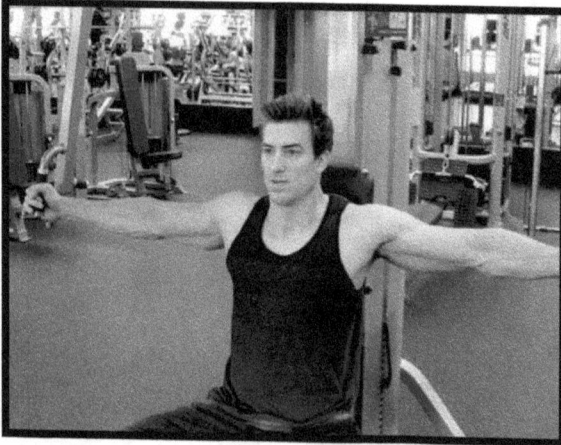

PEC DECK FLYES

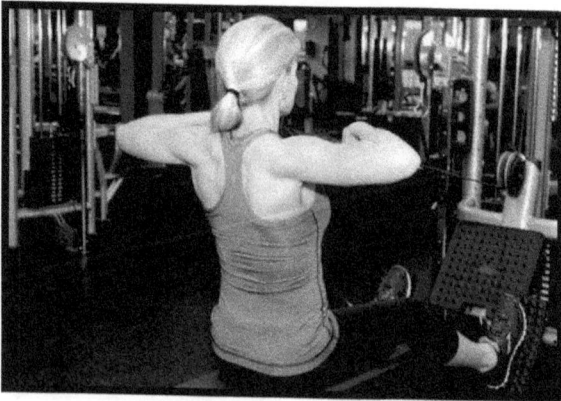

RHOMBOID PULLS TO NECK

supersets on the following exercises, just moving from set to set with less than 2 min. rests.

#2 CHEST & BACK

- 4 x 22-11 Flat Bench Press
- 4 x 22-11 Lat Pulldowns
- 4 x 22-11 Decline Bench press

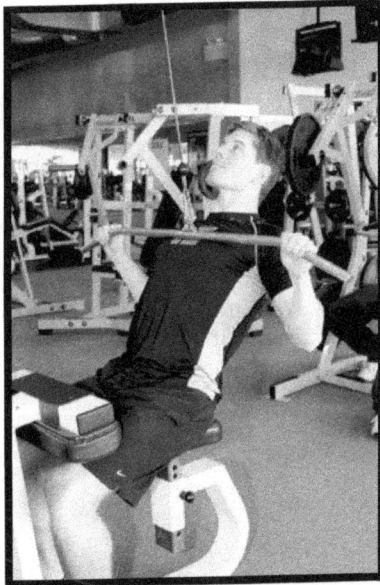

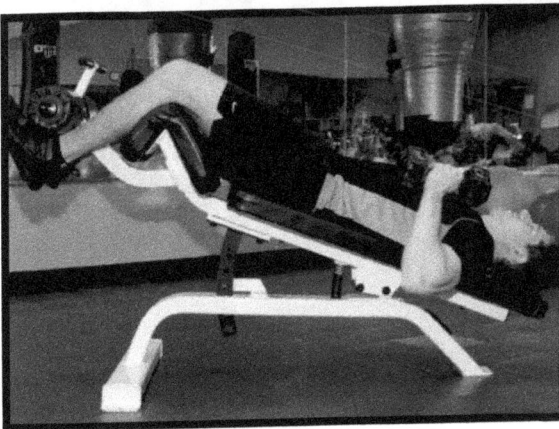

- 4 x 22-11 Seated Pulley Rows
- 3 x 22 Incline Dumbbell Press – knuckles to ribcage
- 3 x 22 each Single Dumbbell Rows

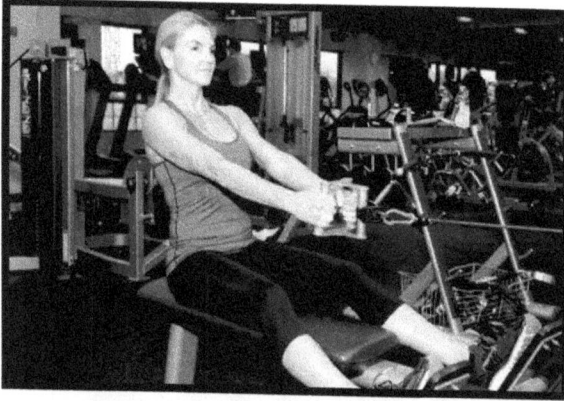

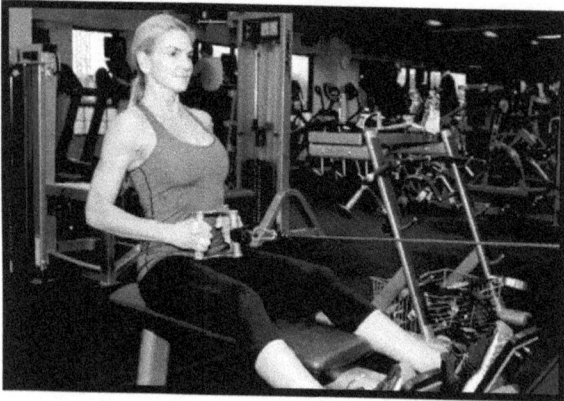

SEATED PULLEY ROWS

#3 CHEST & BACK

- 2 x 11 Pull ups
- 2 x 11 Dips
- 4 x 22-11 Lat Pulldowns
- 4 x 22-11 Smith-machine Bench Press
- 3 x 20 per side Twin T Towers
- 3 x 22 per side Single Seated Pulley Rows
- 4 x 22-11 Dumbbell Flyes
- 4 x 22-11 Seated Pulley Rows

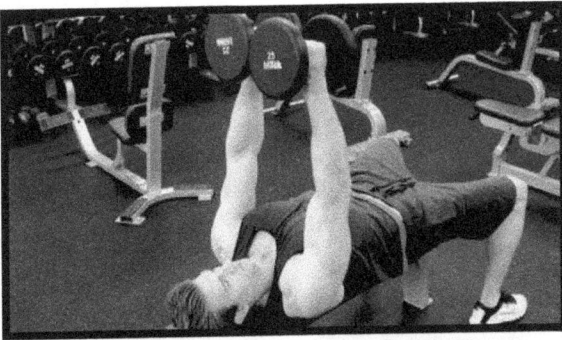

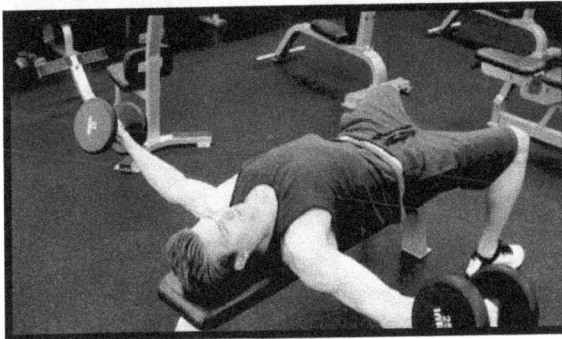

DUMBBELL FLYES

#4 CHEST & BACK

- 3x11 Pullups
- 3x11 Dips
- 4x11 Flat Bench Press
- 4x11 T-bar Rows
- 4x11 Incline Dumbbell Press

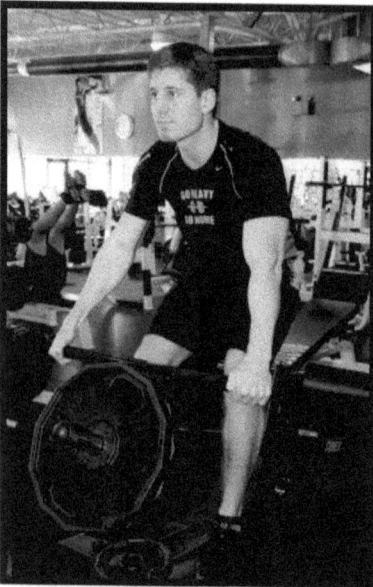

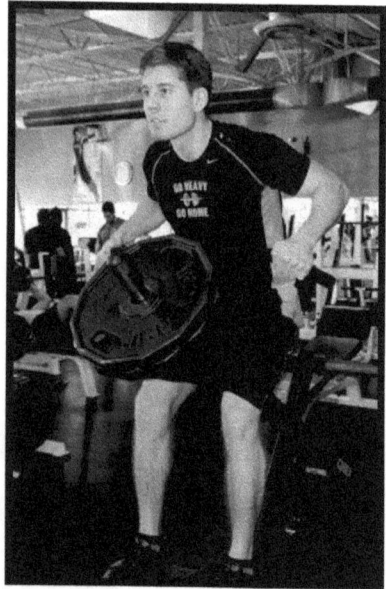

T-BAR ROWS

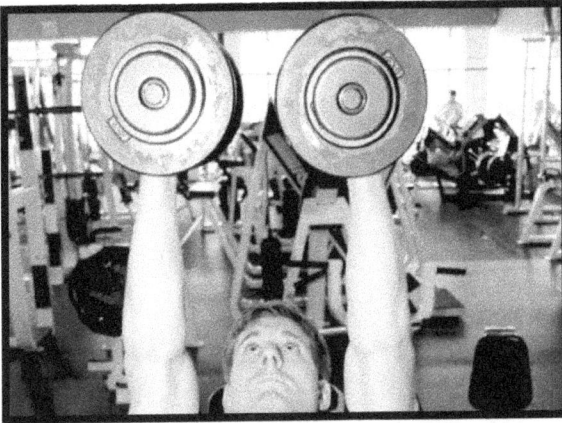

INCLINE DUMBBELL PRESS

- 4x11 Seated Pulley Rows
- 3x22 Decline Dumbbell Flyes
- 3x22 each Single Dumbbell Rows

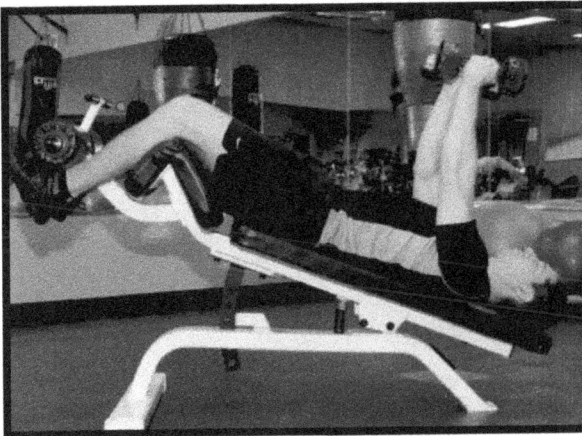

DECLINE DUMBBELL FLYES

#4 CHEST & BACK

- 4x 22-11 Flat Bench Press – bring to bottom ridge of pectorals
- 4x 22-11 Bent-over Barbell Rows – pull to the belly button

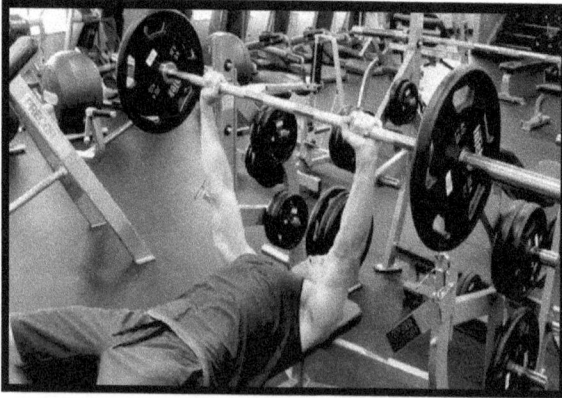

FLAT BENCH PRESS

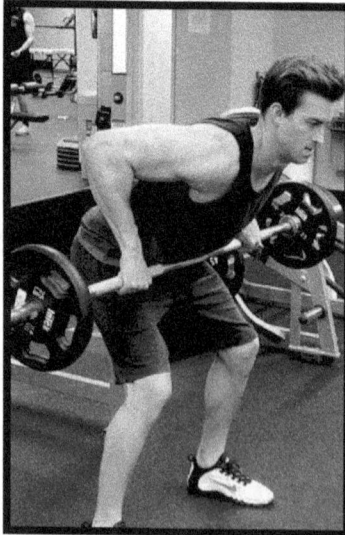

BENT OVER BARBELL ROWS

- 4x 22-11 Incline Bench Press – wide grip, to the top of the chest. Elbows should be down below the bar level to avoid excess stress on the shoulders. Push from under the barbell.

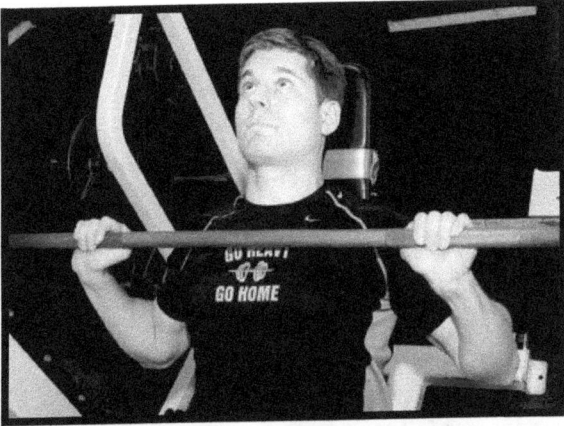

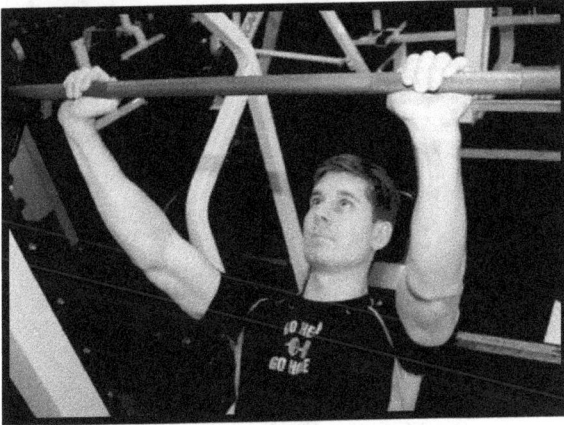

INCLINE BENCH PRESS

- 4x22-11 Pulldowns To Front – below the sternum, to the solar-plexus
- 3x22 Cross Cable Laterals – all done in the low bent-over zone across the mid-chest
- 3x22 Single-arm Dumbbell Rows – keep the back flat, do not roll the shoulder, pull high

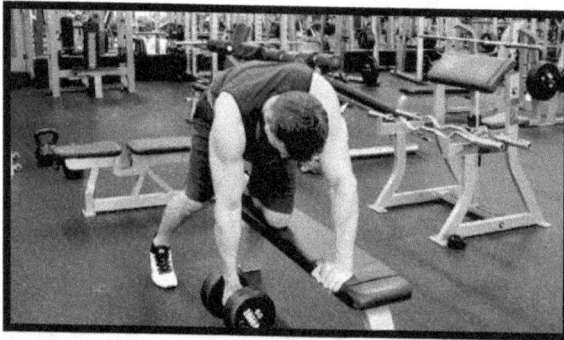

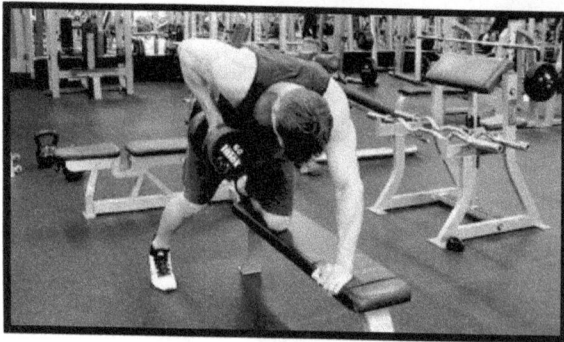

SINGLE ARM DUMBBELL ROWS

#5 CHEST & BACK (no supersets)

- 3 x 22 Cable Crossovers – 3 positions, all the way down; up at 70°; standing straight up
- 3 x 22 Single Handle Cable Rows – on seated pulley machine, draw hand back to ribcage

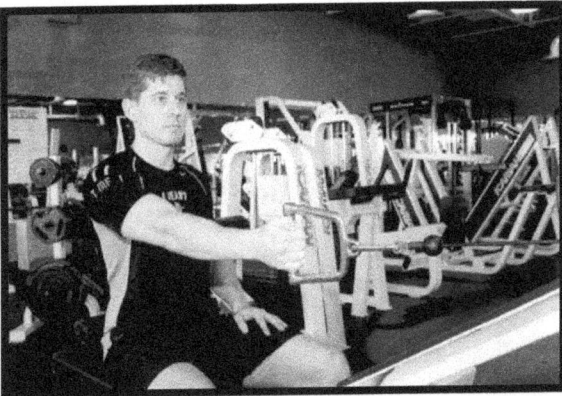

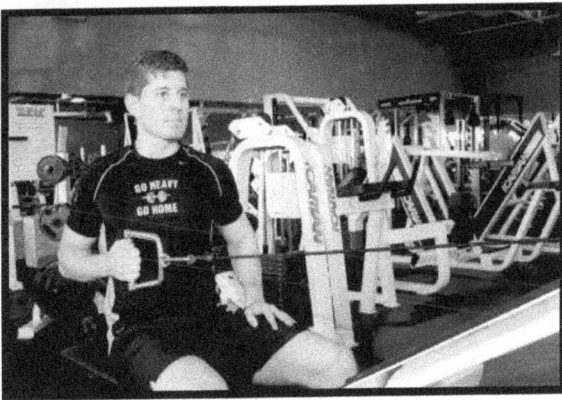

SINGLE HANDLE CABLE ROWS

- 4 x 22-11 Incline Bench Press – bar to collarbone, very strictly
- 4 x 22-11 Pulldowns To Front – hit the collarbone, same spot as the incline press.

These work perfectly along the same range of motion. One is a push, the other a pull; <u>**True Shock And Awe Style.**</u>

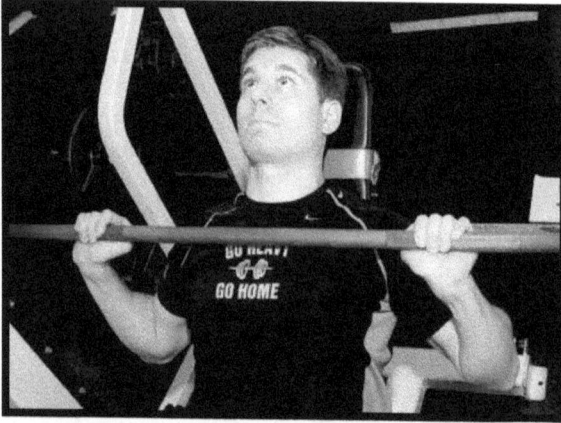

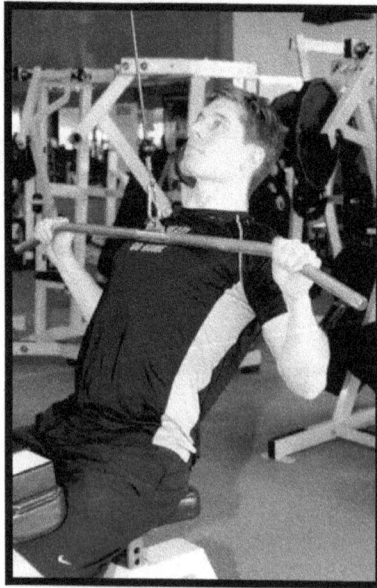

- 4 x 22-11 Flat Bench Flyes – keep an arc in the arms, drop low

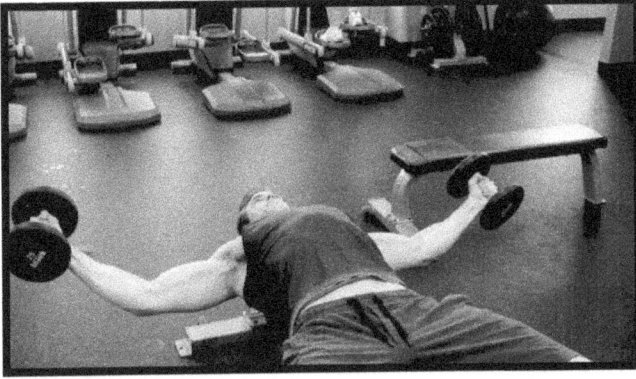

- 4 x 22-11 Barbell Rows – hands wide, pull elbows high

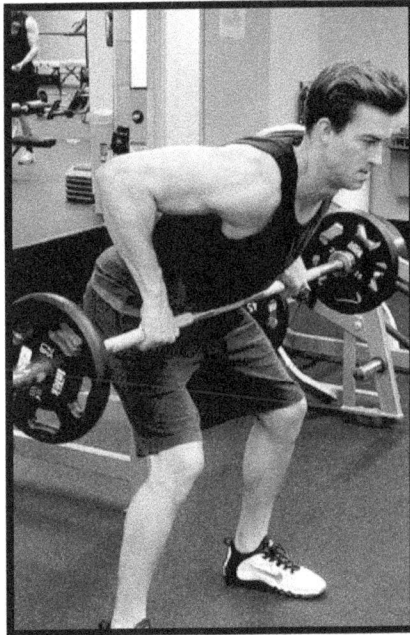

These are great mass building workouts. If you are on limited time, do these to gain overall size on the upper body. Do them every two days, with major Leg workouts on the in-between days. You will be amazed at how large and how lean you will become by following this 4 day regimen. Work on the details later. **This Packs On Muscle!**

SHOCK AND AWE COMBINATION SPECIAL WORKOUTS

#1. LEGS/ CHEST

Legs

• 3 x 22 Stepping Lunges – with barbell, up left, return, up right, return

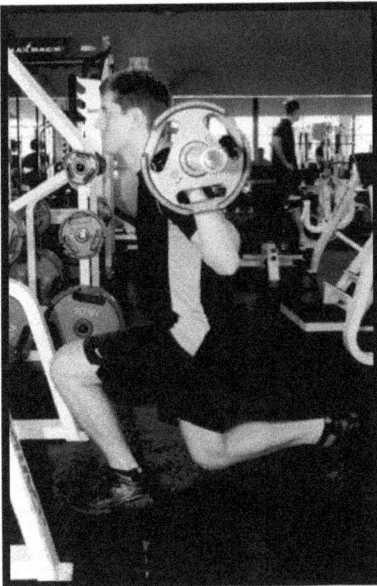

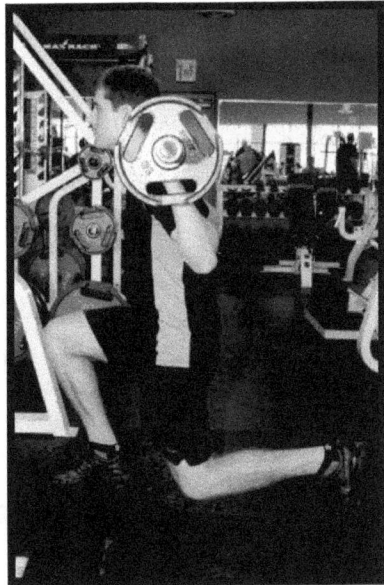

STEPPING ALTERNATING LUNGES

Step forward until the leading and rear knee are at 90°. Keep the back straight, head up and torso tight. Push off the front leg for maximum stimulation to the knee region, but do not let the leading knee go past the toe in the lunge portion.

- 4 x 22-11 Smith Squats - feet forward, back flat, to parallel
- 4 x 22-11 Leg Press

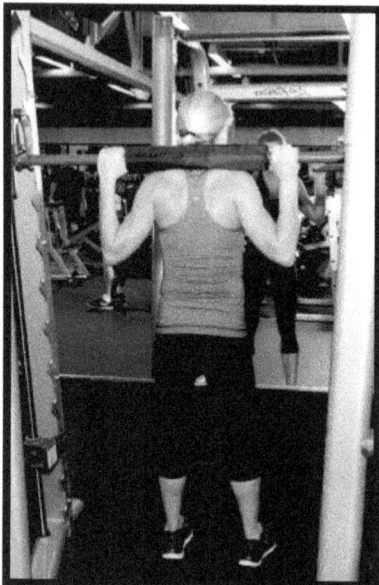

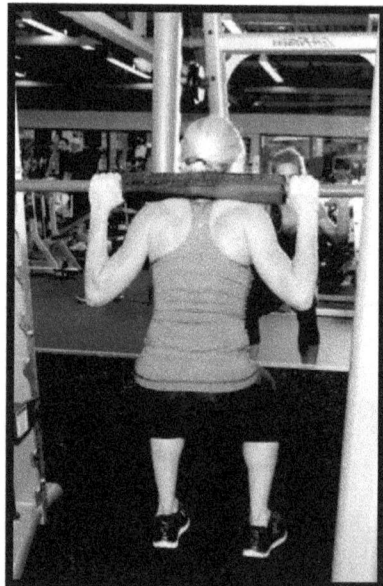

SMITH MACHINE SQUAT

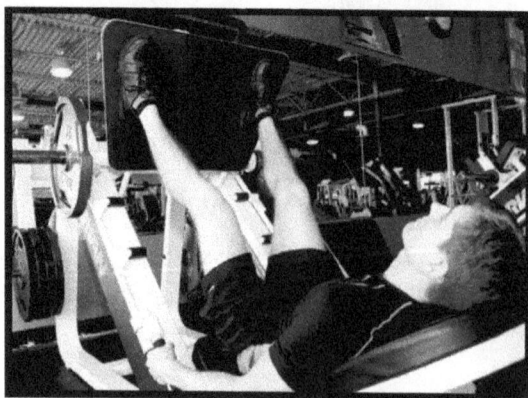

HIGH-WIDE POSITION LEG PRESS

Chest

- 3 x 22 Pec Deck
- 4 x 22-11 Decline Bench Press
- 3 x 20 each side Twin T Towers - on an incline bench, hold two dumbbells over the center of chest, arms extended, always pushing both to center over chest so the tension can be felt along the collarbones. Do 5 left, 5 right, 5 left, 5 right.

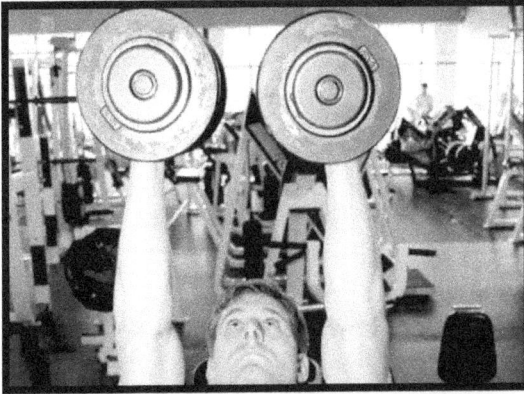

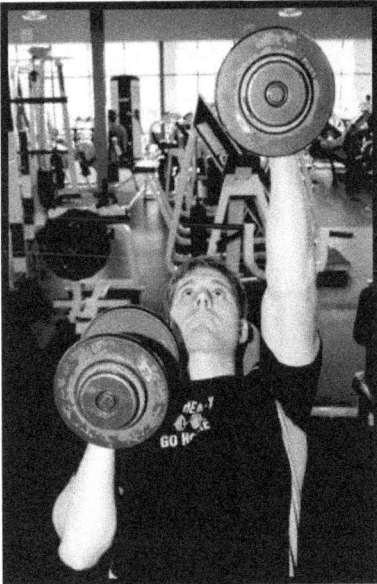

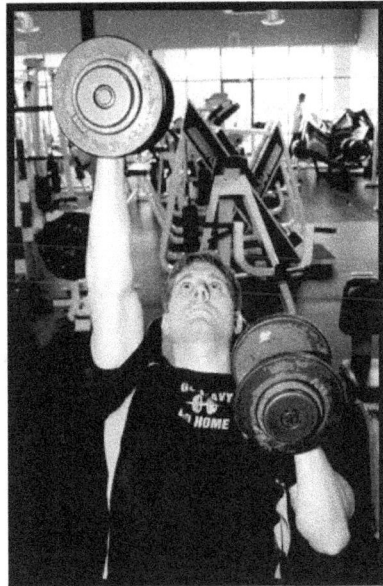

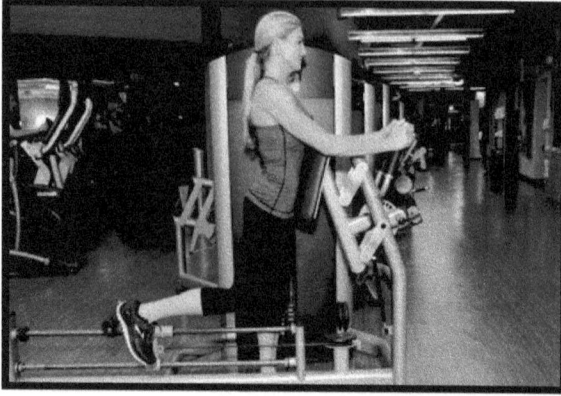

GLUTE PUSHBACKS

#2. LEGS/ SHOULDERS (Intermediate)

<u>Legs</u>
- 3 x 22 Standing Stationary Lunges - with barbell

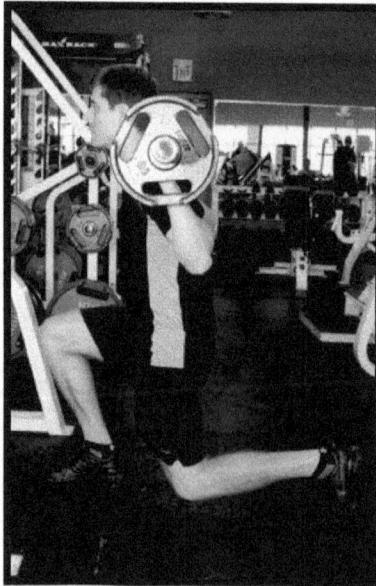

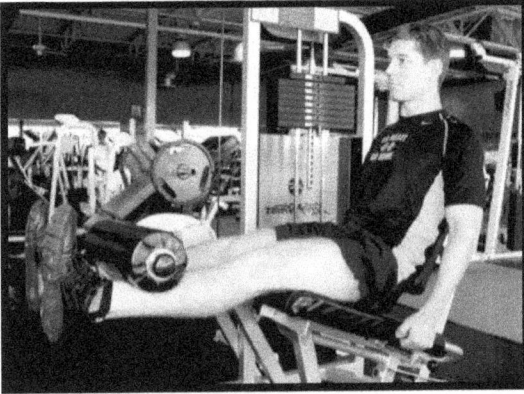

LEG EXTENSIONS

- 4 x 22-11 Leg Extensions
- 4 x 22-11 Leg Curls

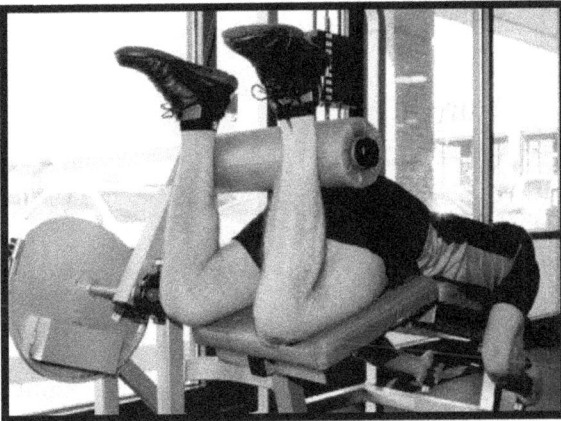

LEG CURLS

Shoulders

- 2 x 22-11 Rear Barbell Press

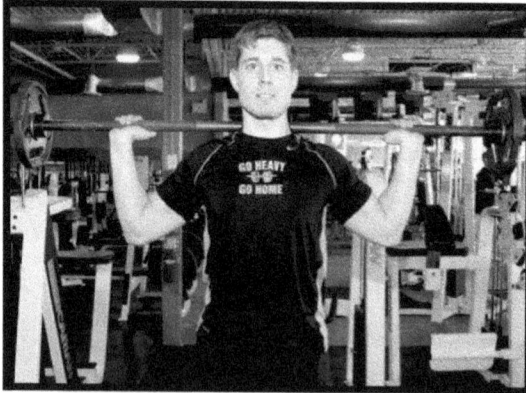

- 2 x 22-11 Front Barbell Press

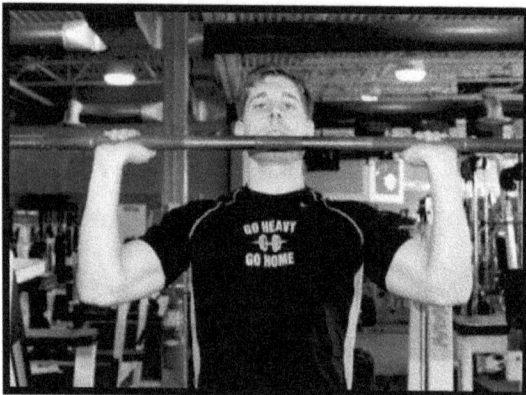

- 4 x 22 Alternate Seated Alternating Dumbbell Press
- 3 x 11 each Side - Front - Rear Dumbbell Lateral Raise

On this Seated Alternating Dumbbell Press be sure to begin with knuckles facing each other in the down position and rotate as you extend to the top of the lift in a corkscrew fashion so the knuckles end up facing the front. This incorporates the front and side deltoid planes.

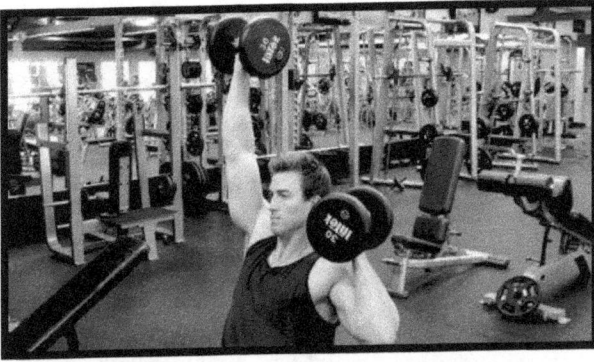

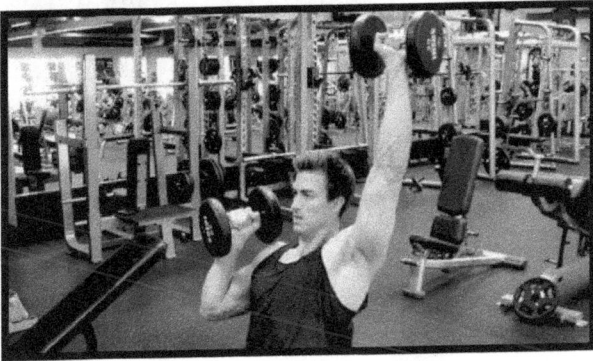

SEATED ALTERNATING DUMBBELL PRESS

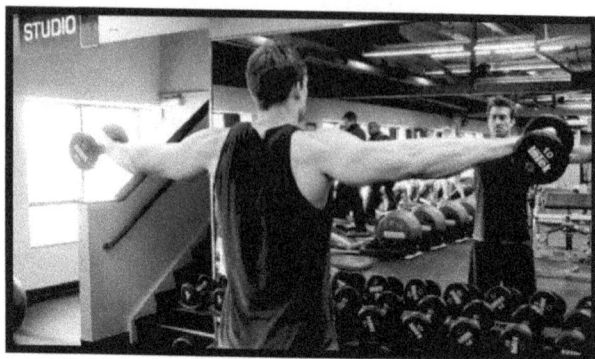

SIDE LATERAL

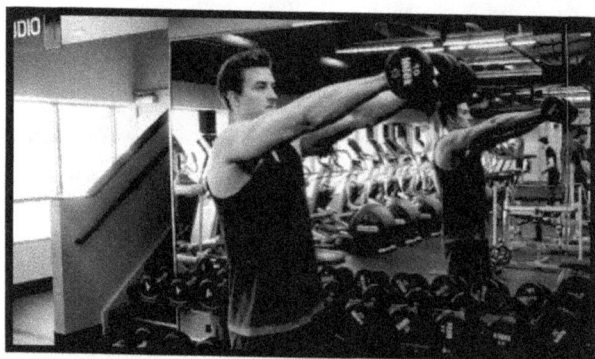

FRONT LATERAL

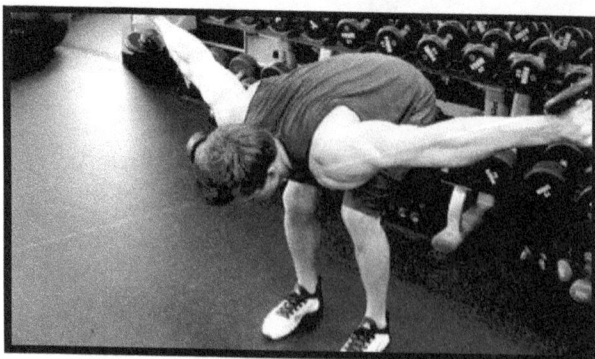

REAR LATERAL

#3. LEGS/ SHOULDERS (Advanced)

<u>Legs - Giant Superset</u>
- 4 x 22-11 Inner Thigh Abductors
- 4 x 11-22 Outer Thigh Adductors

Sit forward in the seat to include the core in the movement. The weight should be adequate to offer enough resistance, but not too much to limit range of motion. Sit up so the core does the stabilizing work, rather than resting on the back cushion.

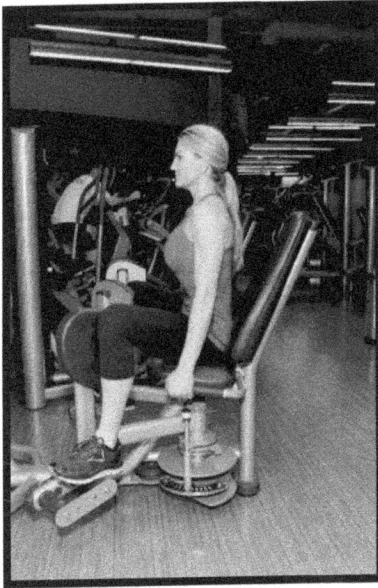

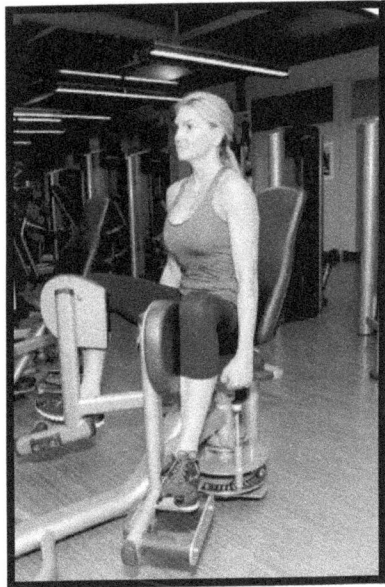

INNER THIGH ABDUCTORS

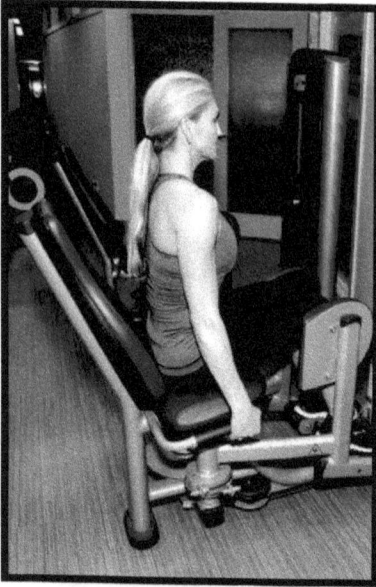

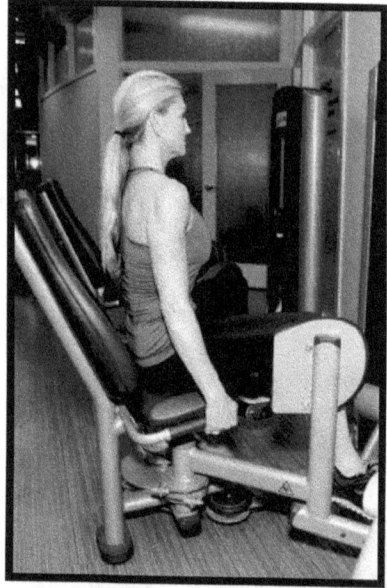

OUTER THIGH ADDUCTORS

- 4 x 22-11 Glute Pushbacks
- 4 x 11-22 Seated Calf Raises

On the Glute Kickback, it is necessary to push through the heel and focus on the hamstring/glute connection by keeping the knee slightly bent, rather than on extending the leg, which flattens out the hamstring and takes the glute out of the movement.

120

On the Seated Calf Raise, change the foot position according to which area of the calf needs most development; toes in to hit outer calves; toes out to hit inner calves; toes straight ahead to hit inner and outer equally.

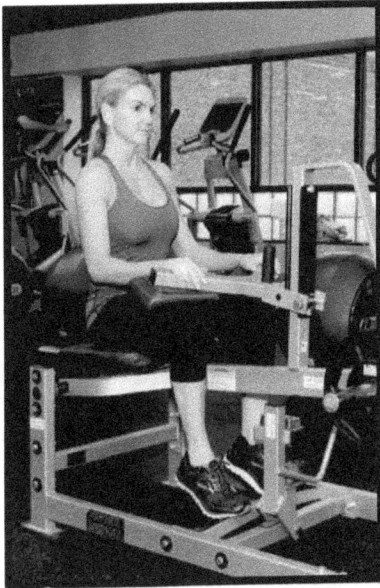

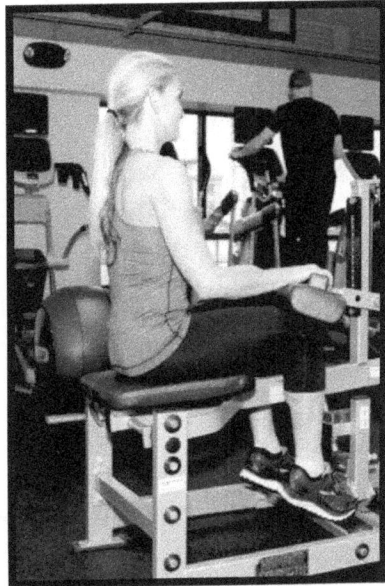

SEATED CALF RAISE

Shoulders – Giant Superset

- 2 x 22 Over and Back Presses on Smith machine
- 2 x 11-22 Behind the Neck Smith presses *superset with*
- 2 x 22-11 Front of Neck Smith presses

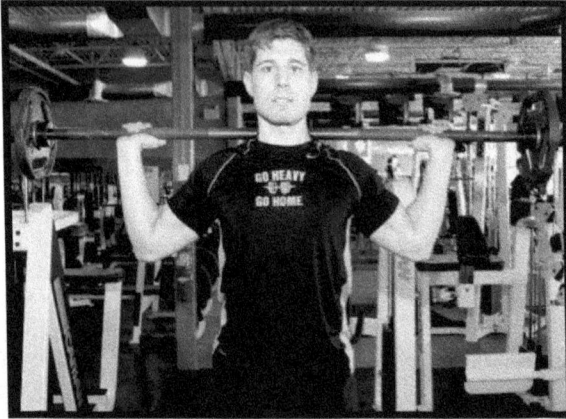

BEHIND THE NECK

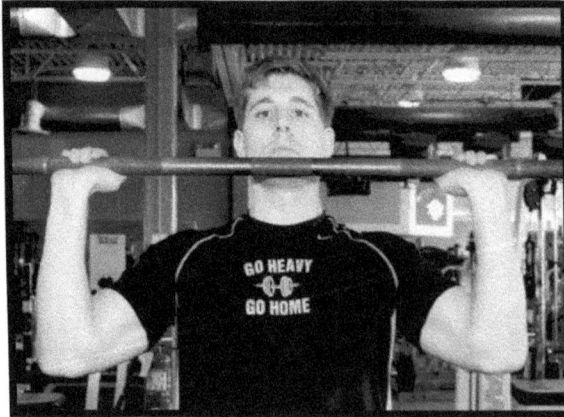

IN FRONT OF NECK

• 3 x 22 Rear Deltoid Barbell Rows to Chin

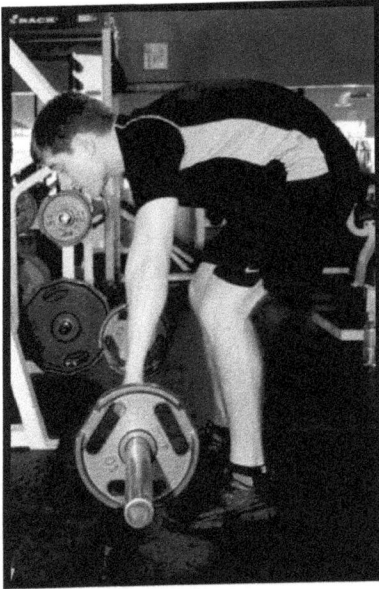

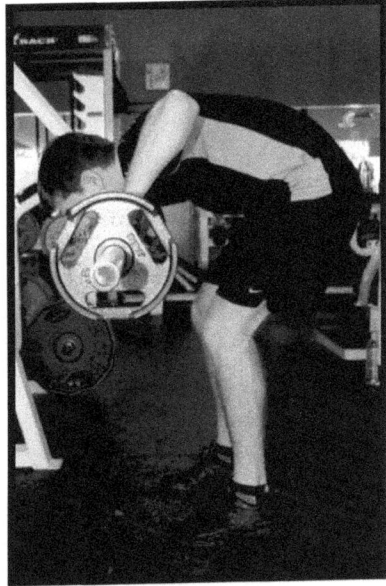

REAR DELTOID BARBELL ROWS

It is crucial to get this movement right so the stress stays on the rear deltoids and not the latissimus. The elbows must be kept forward along the shoulder girdle with a distinct and direct pull to the chin. Let the arms hang loose so the shoulders do the pulling and not the triceps or lats.

• 3 x 11 Dumbbell Side Laterals
• 3 x 11 Barbell Front Laterals

#4. QUICKWORK WHOLEBODY WORKOUT
for SPEED/ STRENGTH/ ENDURANCE

- 6 mins. Jump rope
- 55 pushups

Perform these two moves first, then do all of the following one move after another, in succession, from the Squats to the Lunges, 5x6 each;

- 5x6 squats
- 5x6 cleans
- 5x6 flat benches
- 5x6 rows
- 5x6 dead lifts
- 5x6 dips
- 5x6 directional lunges, no weight

then

- STRETCH

This is a great workout when your time is limited and you want to hit every bodypart, while still getting a good workout.

The Deadlifts should be done with a flat back, feet under the bar, arms fully extended and head up. Lift through the glutes and not the arms or back, lift from the ground up.

The Directional Lunges should be done in a big enough space to allow you to step in this order: Always return to Center

Left forward	return
Right forward	return
Left out	return
Right out	return
Left back	return
Right back	return

This equals one repetition

Until all 6 Repetitions are completed, then go back to Squats

#5. LEGS AND SHOULDERS

- 4 x 22-11 Smith squats
- 4 x 22-11 Lunges
- 3 x 22 Leg extensions
- 3 x 22 Leg curls
- 3 x 22 Standing Alternate Dumbbell Presses
- 3 x 11 each Front, Side, Rear Dumbbell Lateral *superset*
- 11 Smith lunges on 2 risers with 10 lb. plates
- 22 Smith lunges on 1riser with 5 lb. plates
- 33 Smith lunges on 0 risers with 0 plates

You can vary this according to strength and ability.

The higher the step, the better curve you will get at the Glute - Hamstring connection. This delineates the muscles and puts that much sought-after curve at the bottom of the butt, while also lifting it. Done this way, you are doing the hardest work first, and the higher repetitions intensify the burn.

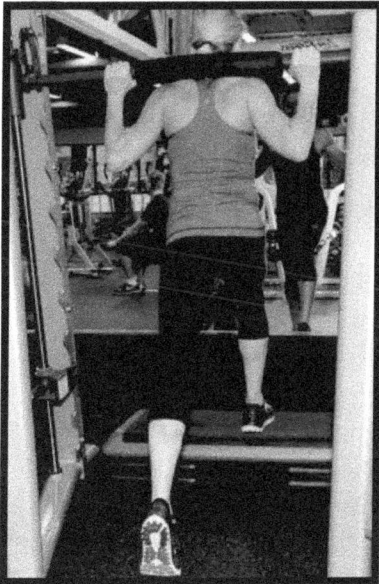

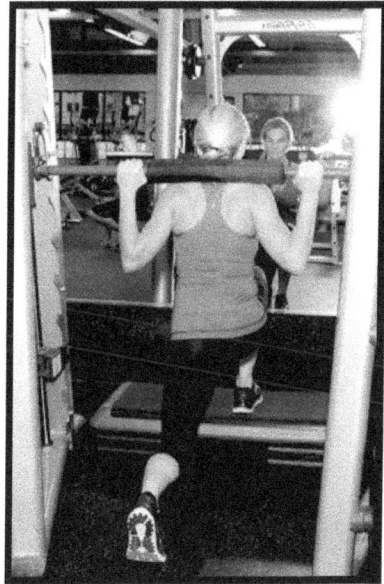

SMITH LUNGES ON RISERS

• 3 x 11 Single Leg Press

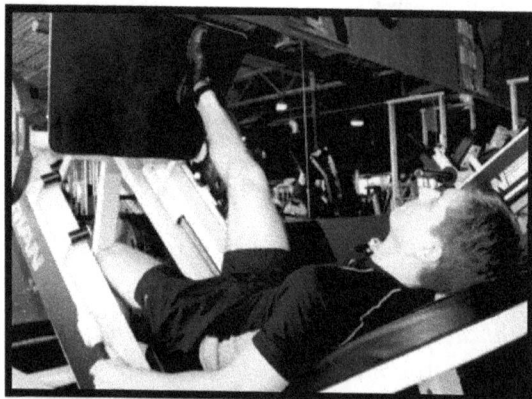

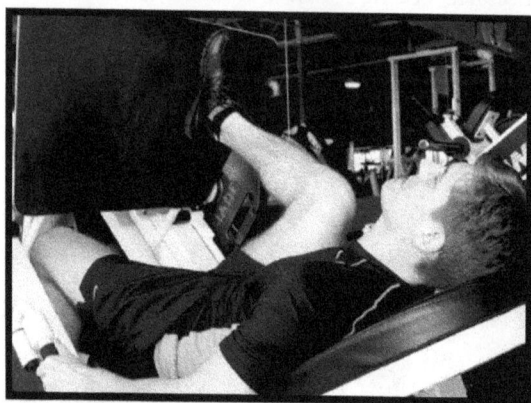

SINGLE LEG PRESS

This is the single best Glute exercise. The foot must be as high as possible on the platform with the toe, knee and shoulder in alignment on the descent. Pull the platform toward the body with full control until the hip pulls off the pad, rather than letting the weight control the drop. Bring in as far toward the shoulder as possible; then forcefully push through the heel to stretch the leg to the return position. Keep the opposite leg extended to avoid being hit by the platform on its descent.

• 3 x 22 Double Leg Press

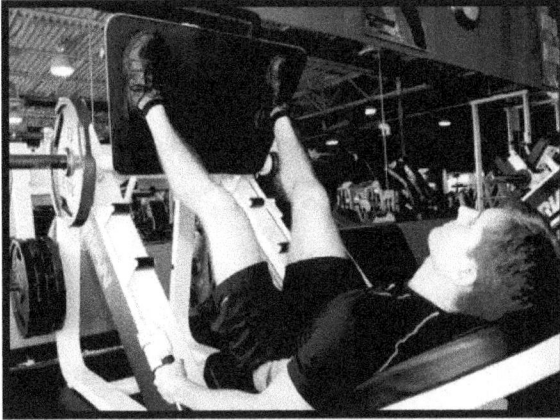

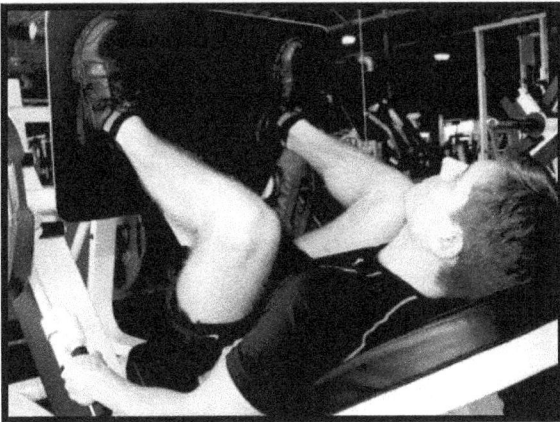

LEG PRESS

To hit different areas of the leg, use various foot positions to get the effect you desire. The higher up the legs are on the platform, the more the hamstrings and glutes will be affected; the further apart, the more the inner thigh is worked. The lower they are on the platform, the more the quadriceps will be activated.

1 x 22 Leg Extensions   *superset with*
1 x 11 Leg Curls
1 x 11 Leg Extensions   *superset with*
1 x 22 Leg Curls
4 x 22 Seated Calf Raises

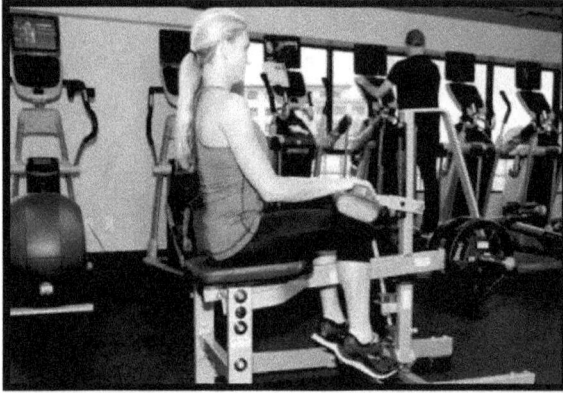

SEATED CALF RAISES

You can try different foot positions with these to activate different sides of the calves; toes pointed in for outer calves; toes pointed out for inner calf; straight ahead for full calves.

#6. LEGS/ CHEST

Legs
- 3 x 22 step lunges
- 4 x 22-11 Smith squats
- 4 x 22-11 leg press

Chest
- 3 x 22 pec deck
- 4 x 22-11 decline bench press
- 4   x   20   each   – Twin   T   Towers

Do not let the simplicity of this workout fool you. It is a very adequate workout when building sheer size or strength. You must cut down the rest time while adding concentration. You can also go pretty heavy since it is not too grueling in regard to many movements or supersets; but you will still get a great pump out of this and be pleased with your results.

#7. ARMS/SHOULDERS WORKOUT

- 3 x 22 Cable Curls   *superset with*
- 3 x 22 Overhead Rope Pulls   *superset with*
- 3 x 22 Barbell Presses

And then one giant Superset
- 3 x 22 Alternating Dumbbell Curls *superset with*

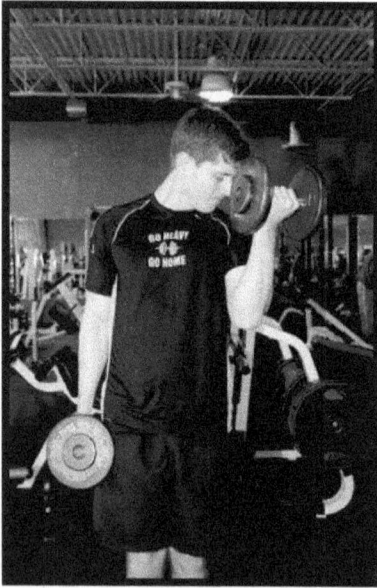

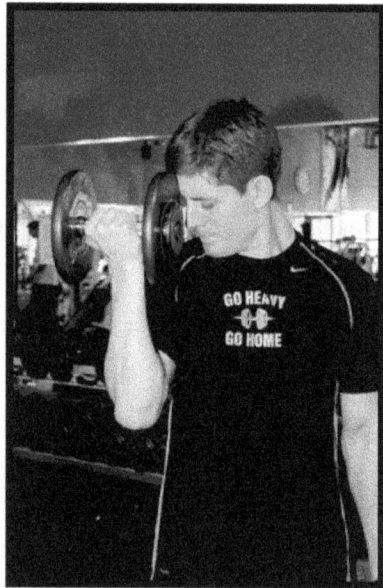

ALTERNATING DUMBBELL CURLS

Be sure to push the inner head of the dumbbell over the peak of the biceps to ensure full stimulation and peak effect to the exercise. It helps to turn your head, both for concentration and to assist in turning the dumbbell over the biceps head.

• 3 x 11 Triceps Skull Crushers   *superset with*

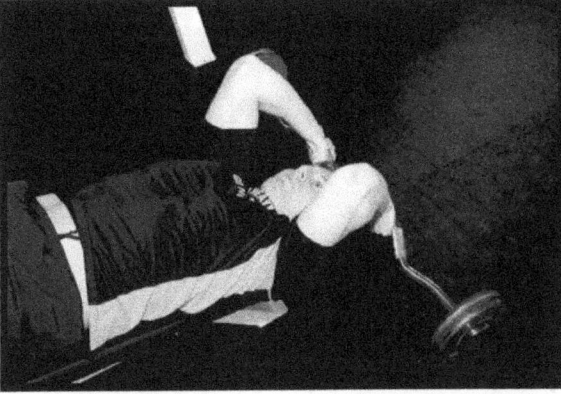

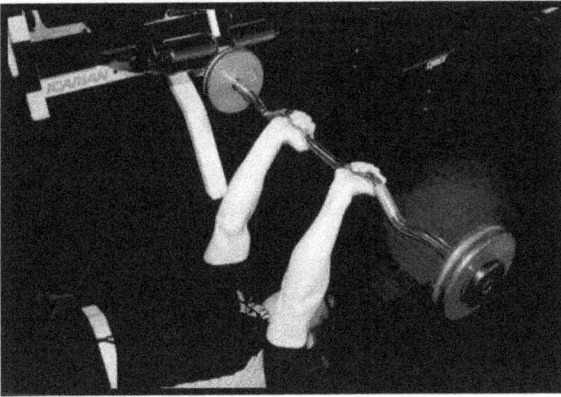

TRICEPS SKULL CRUSHERS

These do not really hit the top of the head, but graze over the peak of the forehead. They can be done with a straight or E-Z Curl bar, which is easier on the wrists than a straight bar.

- 3 x 11 Rear Deltoid Barbell Rows to Chin *superset with*
- 3 x 11 Reverse Handle Triceps Pulldowns *superset with*
- 3 x 11 Single Handle Bicep Curls   *superset with*

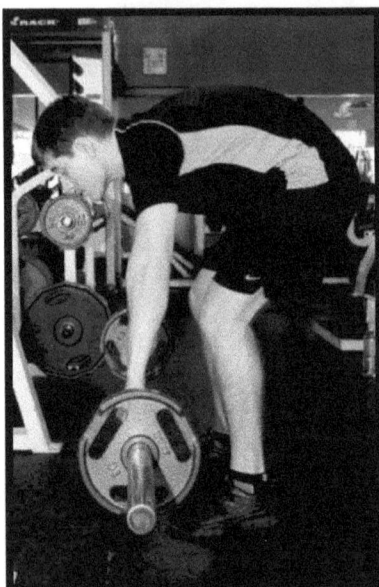

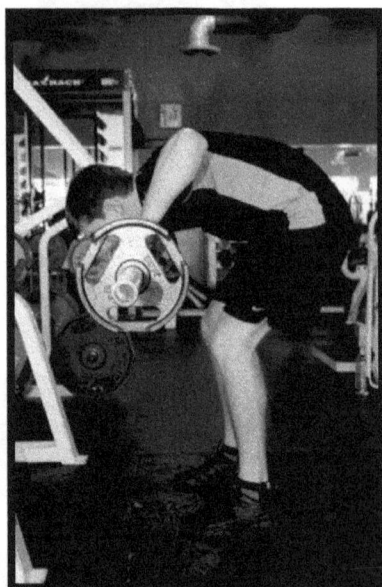

REAR DELTOID BARBELL ROWS

It is crucial to keep the elbows forward in this move, to ensure that the stress goes to the rear deltoids and not the lats. As soon as the elbows drop backward, the latissimus becomes involved.

A good guideline is to keep the elbows over the barbell and pull directly to the chin. If this strictness is too hard, drop the weight until you can perform every repetition in this manner. This is a key bulking movement for the rear deltoids and if you find you are not getting a good burn and immediate results on the first set, you are doing something wrong in its execution.

• 3 x 11 Side Lateral Cable Pulldowns

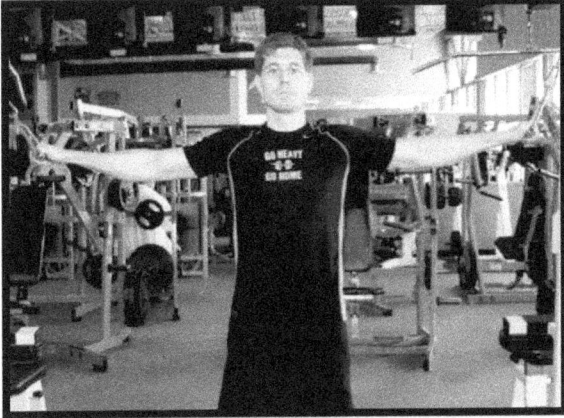

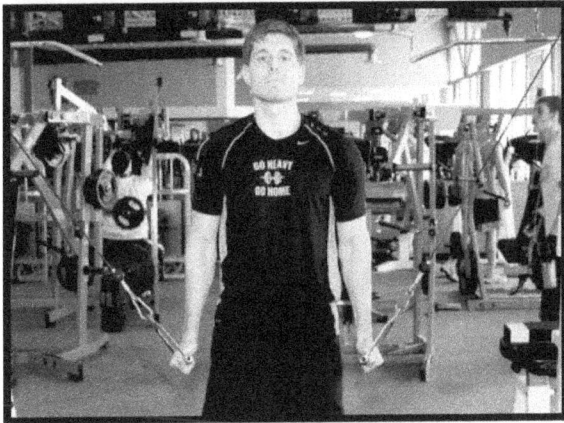

Pull so the little finger of each hand reaches the thigh first and the head stays up, driving the stress to the middle and rear deltoid heads of the shoulders. Stand as straight as possible and hold at the bottom of the movement to accentuate the separation between these heads. Do not use too much weight, but DO use too much form!

SHOCK AND AWE© *Legs*

I'd always had an affinity for leg training. You either like it or hate it, or hate liking it! But either way, to bring balance to the physique, you must train them. Most women enjoy or don't mind training them. They're used to pain. So most of these workouts were made according to women's needs and desires for better legs. I am a Leg Expert; between training 80% women, fitness competitors and designing these for athletes who need incredible endurance, explosive speed or both, these workouts qualify as some of the best for building functional, aesthetically pleasing legs. These are serious routines.

Done in true Shock And Awe fashion, these are truly killer. The high reps seem to be a breeze on the first sets, but once the pump kicks in and the legs barely bend, there's no doubt that these are the most consistently effective workouts for cut, defined legs. The (pain) pleasure lasts for days. Then, when the swelling goes down, you'll discover some new lines peeking out along the hamstrings and quadriceps that weren't there before.

As with all other forms of Shock And Awe Training, Legs are excruciatingly brutal. The upper regions of leg training will have you puking or crying or both, (you sick puppy). If you are experienced in the gym, and you seek out the sickness of a tough challenge, you've found it. Here it is.

Go full into each movement on the warm-ups. The deeper you go, the more you will feel the separations between the front and the back of the legs, the heads of the calves, the hip flexors from the abs, the glutes from the hamstrings. Every workout is worse (or better) than any you'd experienced. Call for the fire department. This burn goes deep and the pleasure of being done is unmatched from any other bodypart workout. Hate me today. Love me tomorrow.

#1 LEGS

• 3 x 22 Smith Step Ups

If you can do these on the first try, all the sets and reps, than you are a bona fide BadAss! These are very tough, and very effective at hitting the glute-hamstring tie-ins. They must be done with excellent form. Keep the knee next to the step, floating, so all the pressure is kept on the top leg. Let the knee descend below the step. Keep the top leg engaged and the back straight throughout.

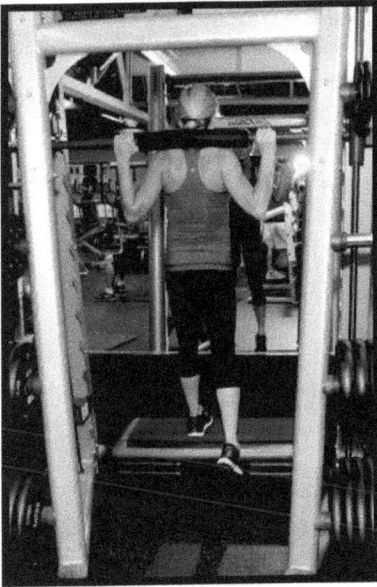

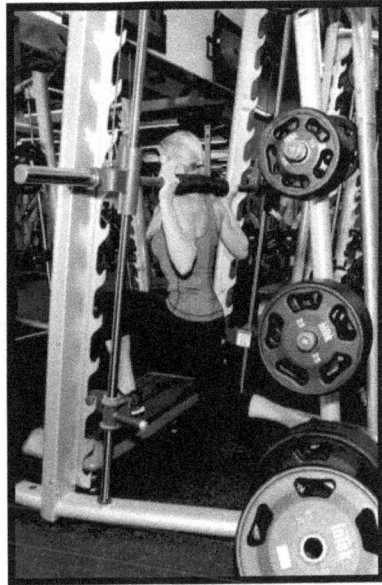

SMITH STEP UPS

• 4 x 22-11 Hack squats

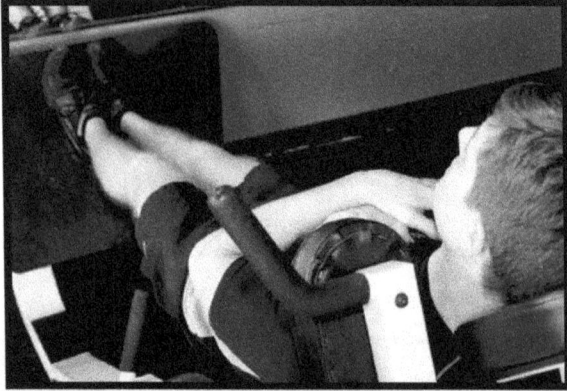

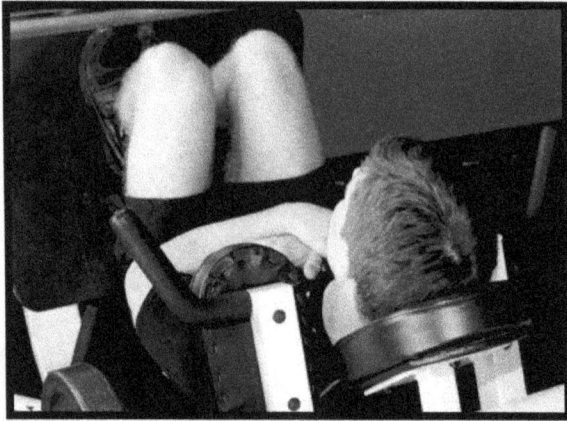

NARROW HACK SQUATS

Be certain to keep the lower back pressed into the pad so the hips do not raise off the bench. Just like the Leg Press, the higher up on the platform, the more the back of the legs get worked; the lower the feet, the more the quadriceps and outer leg get worked. Go light to be able to go low; remember, the hips must go below the knees to engage the glutes.

• 4 x 22-11 Single Leg Press

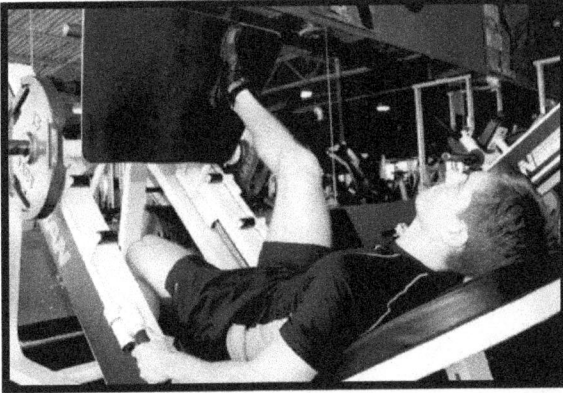

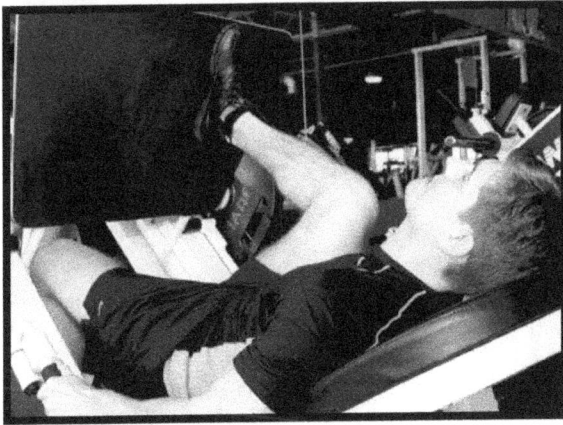

This is the single best Glute exercise. The foot must be as high as possible on the platform with the toe, knee and shoulder in alignment on the descent. Pull the platform toward the body with full control until the hip pulls off the pad, rather than letting the weight control the drop. Bring in as far toward the shoulder as possible; then forcefully push through the heel to stretch the leg to the return position. Keep the opposite leg extended to avoid being hit by the platform on its descent.

• 4 x 22-11 Extensions

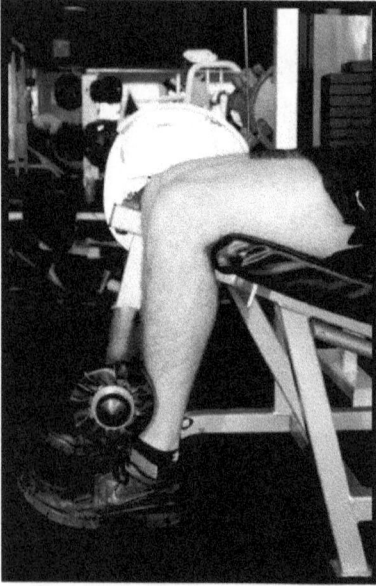

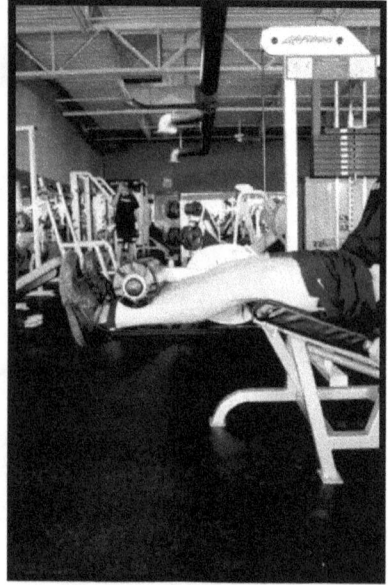

• 4 x 22-11 Leg Curls

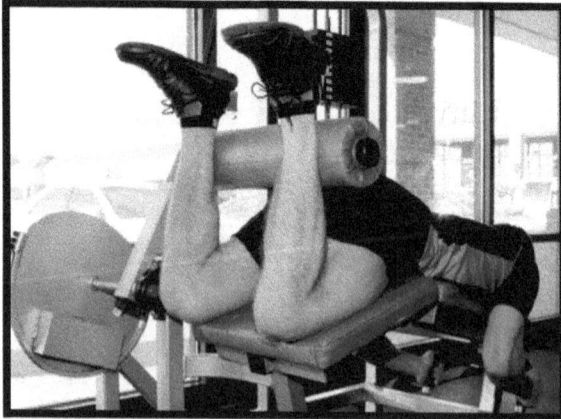

- 6 x 22-11 Seated Calves (3 positions) – toes in, toes out, toes straight ahead *(shown on a leg press for illustration)*

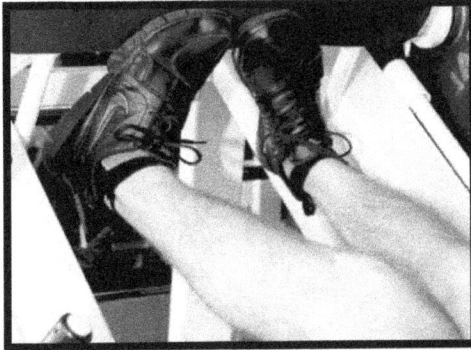

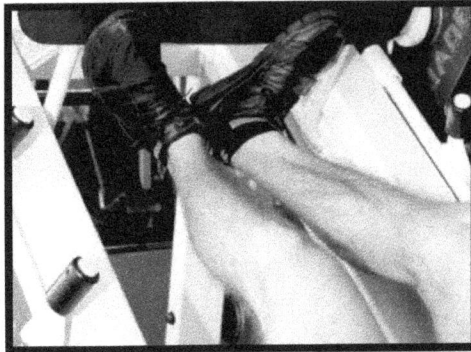

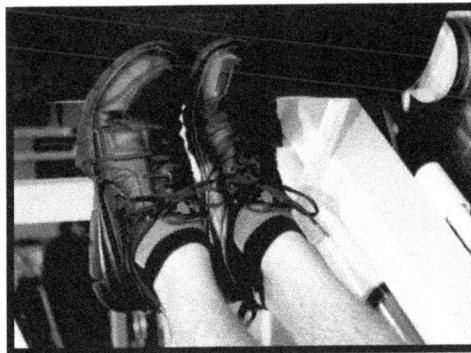

#2 LEGS
3 x 22 Stepping Lunges – with barbell across shoulders

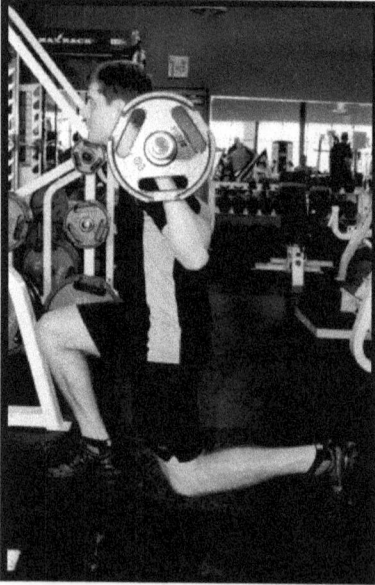

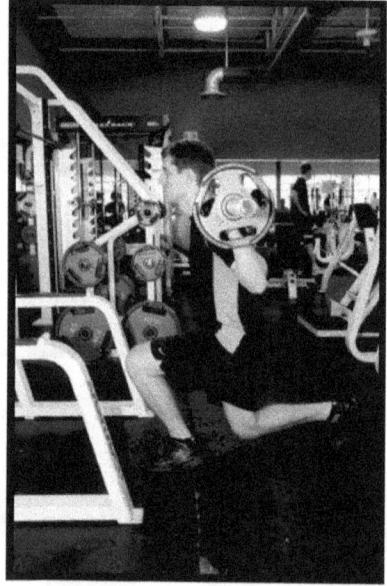

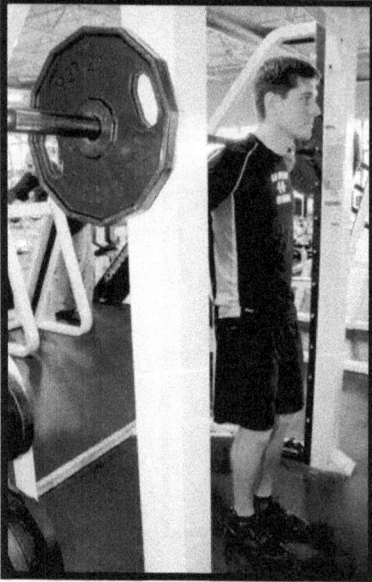

•4 x 22-11 Smith Machine Squats – knees together and forward

- 4 x 22-11 Leg Press - feet low and tight
- 4 x 22-11 Leg Press - feet high and wide

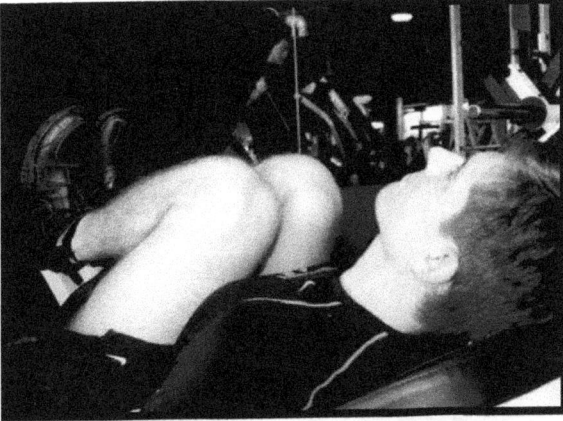

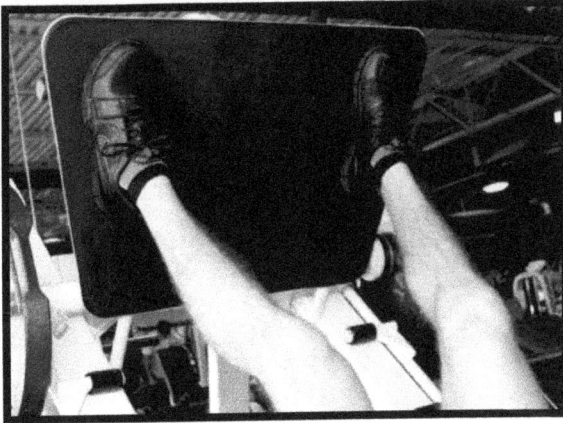

You must put your mind into the muscles here and feel the best foot placement for the type of leg stimulation you want. You can affect every inch, from the hip flexors to the glutes, from the quadriceps to the hamstrings. Learn what best suits your goals with various foot placements and stick with it until you achieve your desired outcome.

• 4 x 11 Stiff Leg Deadlift – preferably off a riser

Raise the head at the top of this movement and pull the body back so the shoulders return over the hips. At the low end, reach toward your shoelaces and keep the bar close to the legs.

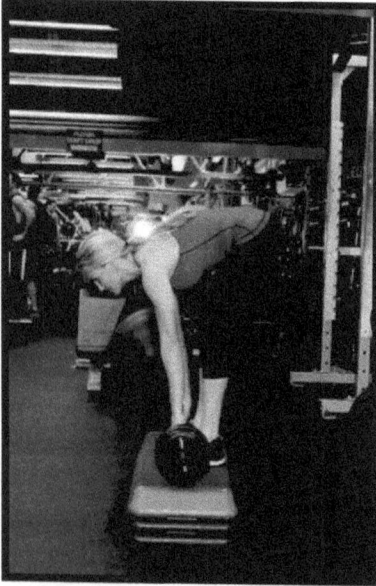

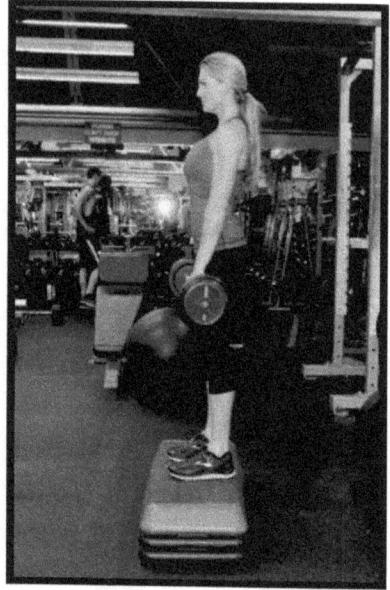

STIFF LEG DEADLIFT

- 4 x 22-11 Leg Extensions   *superset with*
- 4 x 11-22 Leg Curls

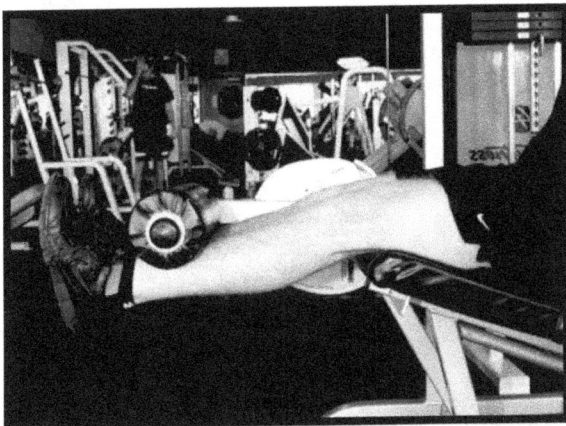

LEG EXTENSIONS

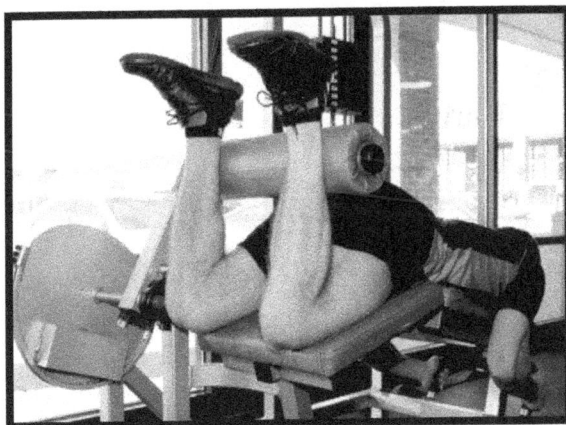

LEG CURLS

• 4 x 22-11 Leg Press Calf Raise

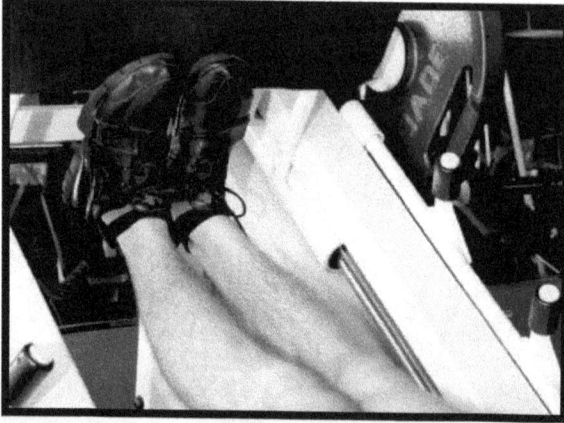

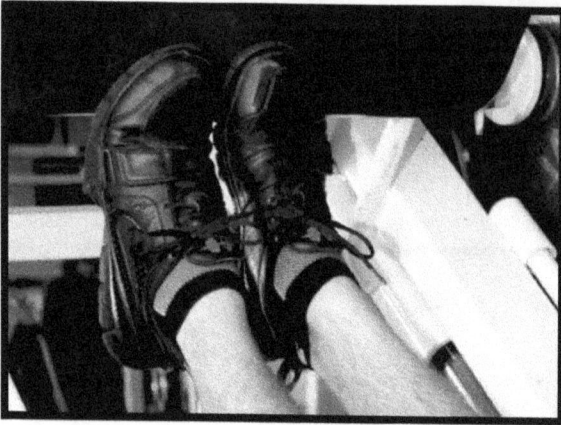

Your calves need much weight to stimulate growth. You lift your body with one foot, with each step you take, all day. So the amount of weight you use must at least START with your actual bodyweight. But work up to it. Never compromise form.

#3 LEGS

- 3 x 22 Smith Step-ups
- 4 x 22-11 Single Leg Press
- 4 x 22-11 Leg Curl
- 4 x 11 Stiff Leg Dead Lift

- 4 x 22 Leg Press Calves 3 positions – in, out, straight and your preference for attention   *superset with*
- 4 x 11 Seated Calves

#4 LEGS

- 4 x 22-11 Leg Curls
- 4 x 11 Heavy Deadlifts
- 3 x 11, 11, 22 Leg Press - single, single, double;
- 4 x 22-11 Squats – freebar, pushing to double the weights on the lower reps

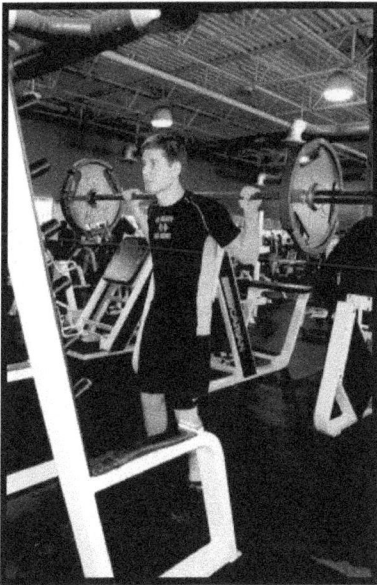

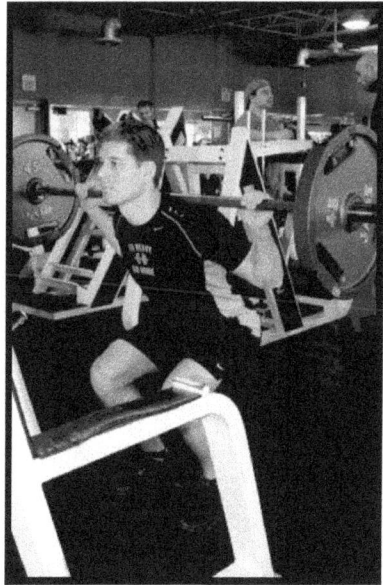

• 4 x 22-11 Smith Lunges – these are stationary lunges, repetitions are for each leg

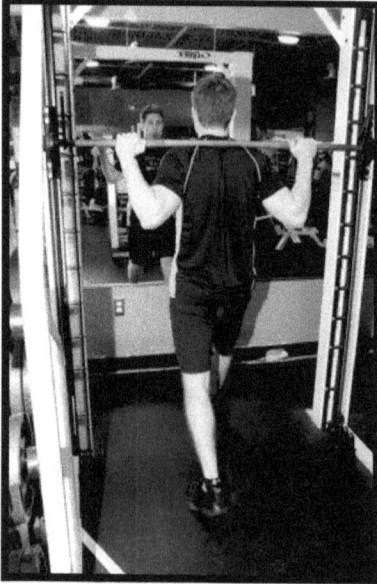

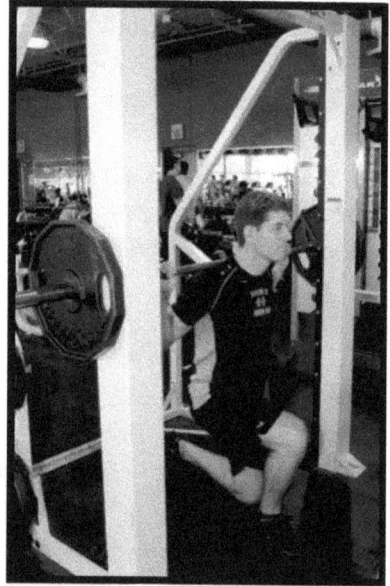

By using the Smith machine for this movement, you lock in form and create a deep groove on the outside separation of the legs, between the hamstrings and quads; and the inner thigh definition, each time you perform them. Keep the back straight and the back knee directly under the bar, forming perfect 90° angles for both legs.

• 6 x 22-11 Seated Calves – two sets in each position; toes in, toes out, toes straight

#5 LEGS

CAUTION:This is possibly the hardest Leg workout routine of all.

- 3 x 11, 22, 33 Smith Drop Lunges - drop riser and weight as reps increase, #each leg
- 11 Smith lunges on 2 risers with 10 lb. plates
- 22 Smith lunges on 1riser with 5 lb. plates
- 33 Smith lunges on 0 risers with 0 plates

You can vary this according to strength and ability.

The higher the step, the better curve you will get at the Glute - Hamstring connection. This delineates the muscles and puts that much sought-after curve at the bottom of the butt, while also lifting it. Done this way, you are doing the hardest work first, and the higher repetitions intensify the burn.

SMITH DROP LUNGES

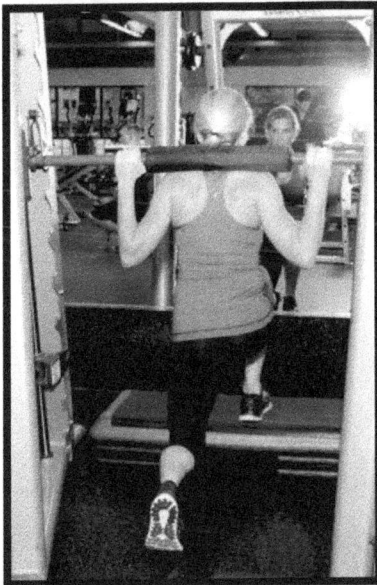

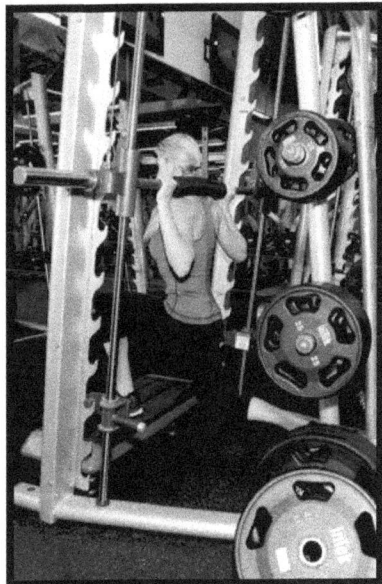

• 4 x 22-11 Low-Zone Squats – on a Smith, everything below parallel is low-zone, stay down

The Low Zone Squat is fantastic for building explosive power and speed for quick-directional sports like hockey and basketball; but also an epic butt builder for physique sports. The whole focus must be kept on staying as low as possible, below parallel, the whole set.

The push comes from the glutes and hamstrings with the heels firmly planted and the push from the tailbone outward, forcing the whole body backward from the top of the gluteus, to the backs of the knees. Stay in the Low Zone, below parallel, the whole set.

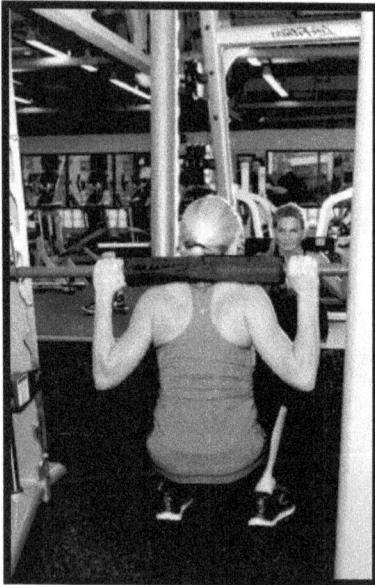

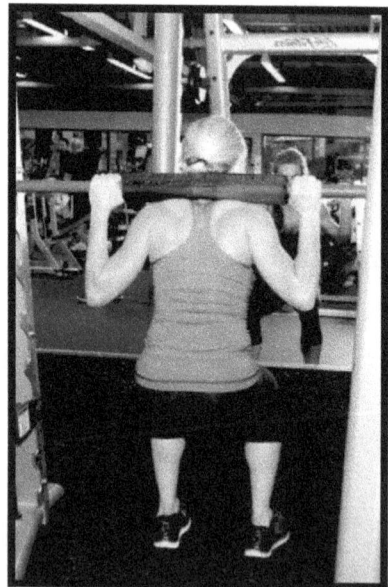

LOW ZONE SQUATS

4 x 11 Squats
4 x 22-11 Hack Squats
4 x 11,11,11,22 Leg Extensions
4 x 22-11 Standing Calves Raises – toes in straight position; deep down, high up, hold

#6 LEGS

- 4 x 22-11 Leg Curls
- 4 x 11 Deadlifts
- 3 x 11,11,22 Leg Press - single, single, double – rest only when adding weight
- 4 x 22-11 Squats
- 4 x 22-11 Smith Lunges - these are stationary lunges, repetitions are for each leg

#7 LEGS

- 3 x 22 Stepping Lunges with Barbell
- 4 x 22-11 Smith Squats
- 4 x 22-11 Leg Press

4 x 22-11 Leg Extensions   *superset with*
4 x 11-22 Leg Curls

#8 LEGS

- 4 X 22-11 Step ups
- 4 X 22-11 Low Zone Squats
- 3 x 22 each Glute Pushbacks on Buttblaster

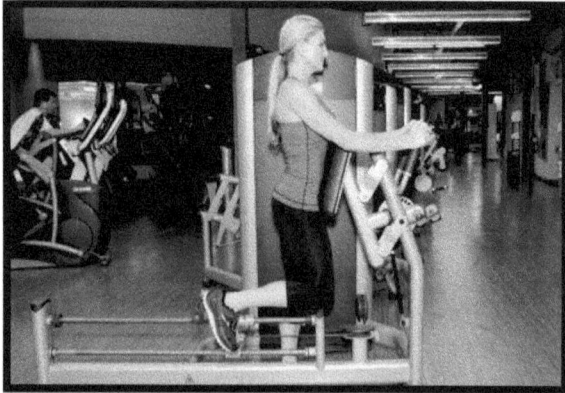

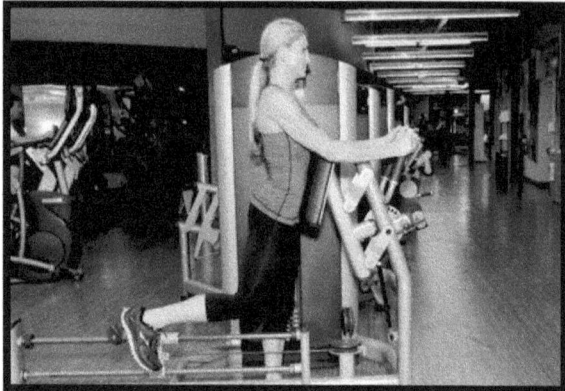

- 4 x 11 each Single Leg Curl
- 4 x 11 Stiff Leg Deadlifts
- 4 X 22 Standing Calves

This is one of the toughest leg workouts on the list, due to the sheer volume of weight, high repetitions and various movements.

#9 LEGS

- 4 x 22-11 Smith Squats
- 4 x 22-11 Leg Press
- 3 x 22, 11, 22 Leg Extensions
- 3 x 11, 22, 11 Leg Curls

A favorite go-to workout when you don't really want to think about legs, but just want to get in there and get them done. It is very effective, highly stimulating and a killer as long as you pay strict attention to form and weights.

The following workout is a tougher , more challenging routine, but also a good, basic, go-to workout on a regular basis.

#10 LEGS

- 3 x 22 Directional Lunges

The Directional Lunges should be done in a big enough space to allow you to step in this order: Always return to Center

Left forward	return
Right forward	return
Left out	return
Right out	return
Left back	return
Right back	return

Until all 6 Repetitions are completed

- 4 x 22-11 Barbell Squats
- 4 x 22 each Single Leg Press
- 3 x 22 Leg Press Calves

3 x 11 Leg Curls   *superset with*
3 x 22 Extensions

#11 LEGS

- 4 x 22-11 Leg Extensions – feet together, knees and toes pointed forward, not outward
- 4 x 11-22 Leg Curls – legs together, pulling straight up, not to the sides
- 4 x 22-11 Hamstring Crunch – hamstring pulldown apparatus, pull heels all the way back

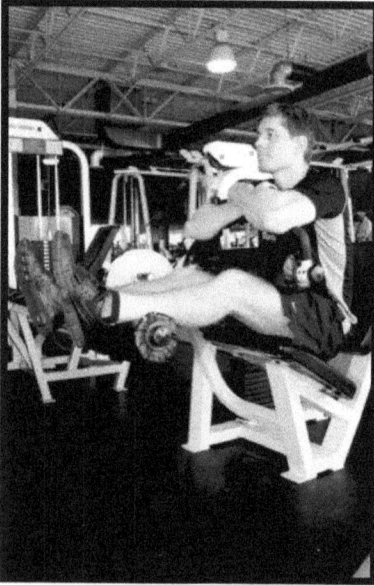

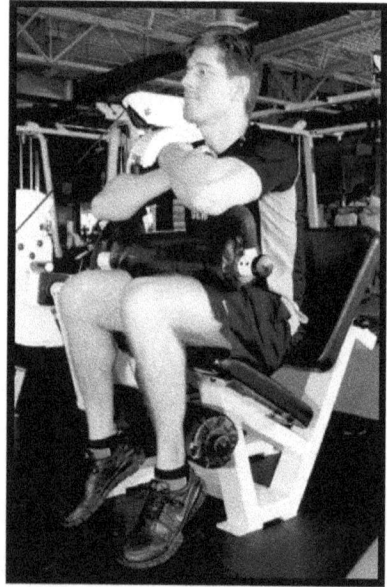

HAMSTRING CRUNCH

- 4 x 11-22 Standing Calves
- 3 x 11 Front Cable Pulls – cuff attached to ankle, smooth, steady pull to front
- 3 x 11 Side Single Cable Raises – cuff attached to ankle, outer leg pulls to outside
- 4 x 22-11 Seated Press

#12 LEGS

- 6 Min Warm-up – some type of cardio, enough to raise your heart rate
- Stretch
- 3 x 11, 22, 33 Smith Drop Lunges - drop riser and weight as reps increase, #each leg
- 4 x 22 Squats - adding weight each set
- 4 x 11 Single Leg Press - deep into the glutes, foot high, ball of foot off
- 6 x 22 Calve Raises on Block or Step – no weight, two sets each of 3 foot positions
- 3 x 22 Abs EACH   Leg Lifts, Scissors Kicks, Crunches, Crossovers

#13 QUICKIE-MINI-LEGS

- 4x11 Squats - go heavy, but deep is more important than heavy
- 4x11 Leg Press - Start with weight you left off at for squats
- 3x11 Stiff Leg Deadlifts – the goal is to touch the tops of the shoelaces with the bar

#14 INNER THIGH EXCLUSIVE

- 3 x 22 Plie' Hack Squats – toes pointed out, sit deep into seat, keep back straight
- 4 x 22-11 Single Leg Press
- 4 x 22-11 Plie' Press (or Smith Squat Plie')
- 4 x 22-11 Inner/ Outer thigh machines – sit up straight and don't lean in or back
- 6 x 11 Seated Calves

#15 SINGLE LEGS

- 3 x 22 Step Ups
- 4 x 11 Single Leg Squat
- 4 x 22-11 Butt Blasts
- 11, 11, 22 Single/ *then* Double Leg Press
- 11, 11, 22 Single/ *then* Double Leg Curl
- 11, 11, 22 Single/ *then* Double Standing Calves

JUST CALVES

- 4x11 Seated Calf Machine
- 4x11 Standing Calf Machine
- 3x22 Off the Edge of a Step - held at high and low positions, no weight

BIG TIME CALVES

- 4 x 22-11 Standing Calf Machine

superset with

- 4 x 11-22 Seated Calf Machine

superset with

- 4 x 22-11 Leg Press Calves

SHOCK AND AWE© SHOULDERS

When training the shoulders in this *Shock And Awe©* System, you can move quickly from one deltoid head to the other – posterior, anterior, medial – because they are relatively small muscles that fatigue quickly but also recuperate quickly, so that when you're done with one movement on one plane, the next plane is ready for a subsequent set.

The most neglected and the most important for people to focus their training on are the posterior, or rear deltoids. They are the smallest of the three heads and are often neglected or not given equal attention due to the many movements typically done for the shoulders which stimulate the anterior and medial heads. When the rear deltoids are prominent, the whole shoulder looks better, the posture looks better, and the shoulder girdle is more equally balanced in both strength and aesthetics.

It makes sense to prioritize this muscle group and hit it first in workouts, but the whole key is finding correct exercises to isolate and stimulate these rear deltoids. The best one for direct impact are Barbell Rows to Chin. The technique for doing these is extremely important and when it's mastered, because of the relative small size of the muscle, allows quick gains in a short period of time. There is nothing like it.

Many of these workouts are similar, but due to the variations on the exercise order and the numbers of sets and reps, each workout gives a different result. Try two or three in rotation and notice which will bring you the pump and stimulation you are looking for. The shoulders need much attention from many angles for full depth, without getting too bulky or chunky and uneven in development.

BARBELL ROWS TO CHIN

Bend at the waist with the knees slightly bent. The back must stay flat for the entire movement. Grasp the barbell with a wider than shoulder grip. Pull it up in a straight line to the chin, forcing the elbows forward so you feel the movement along the trapezius and neck as well as the deltoids. Extend fully toward the floor and repeat for the prescribed repetitions. Make every rep the same as the previous, with very, very strict attention to form that can never waver. Keep forcing the elbows forward and pulling the bar all the way to the chin, not the neck, or collarbones, but to the chin. You want to feel the pull across the shoulder girdle from left to right deltoid across the trapezius and neck, while the back stays flat and the elbows stay forward.

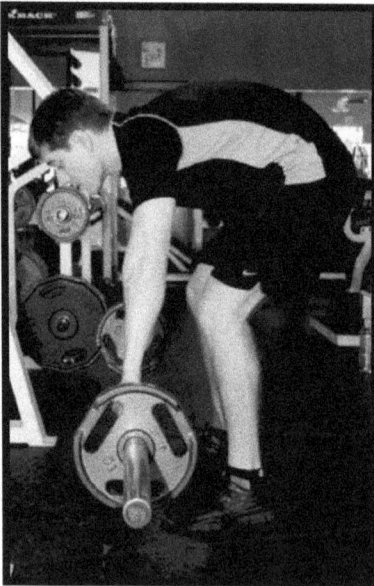

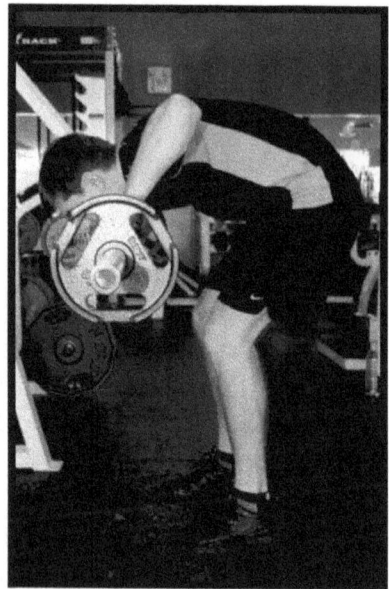

BARBELL ROWS TO CHIN

#1 SHOULDERS

- 33-22-11 Shrugs - back to the bar, fingers point backwards. Begin with lowest weight and work up to heaviest.

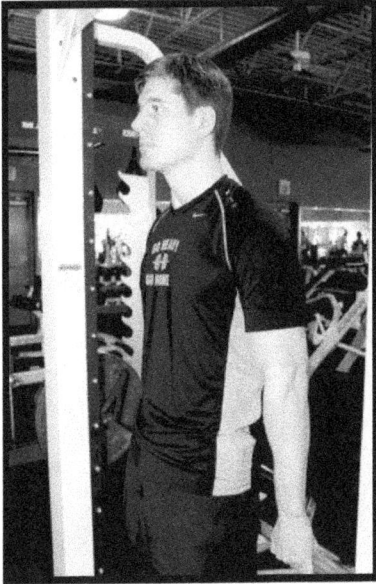

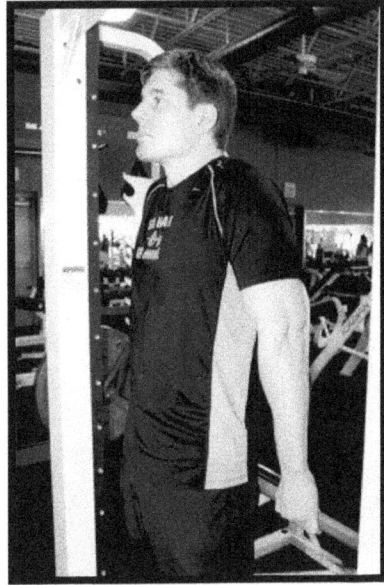

These shrugs work the trapezius muscles, the triangular muscles which bridge the upper shoulder area.

By having the fingers face away from the body, you put emphasis on the rise at the back of the body, accentuating the height of the trapezius. It's important in both planes of movement to keep the elbows locked and use the hands as hooks, pulling the shoulders up toward the ears.

By having the fingers face forward, standing behind the bar, the thickness of the front edge of the trapezius is accentuated. Both grips need to be utilized in order to get as much size out of these muscles as possible.

- 11-22-33 Shrugs - facing bar, fingers forward, pull upward. Use the heaviest weight here and come back down to lightest.

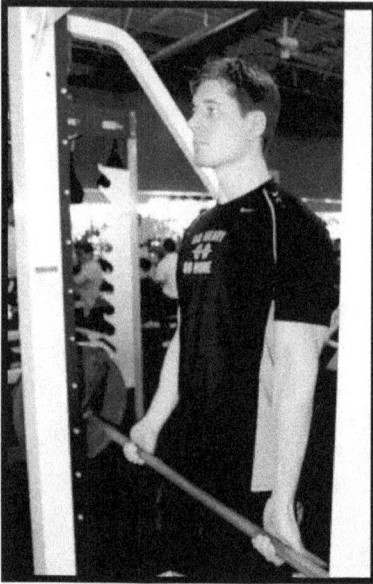

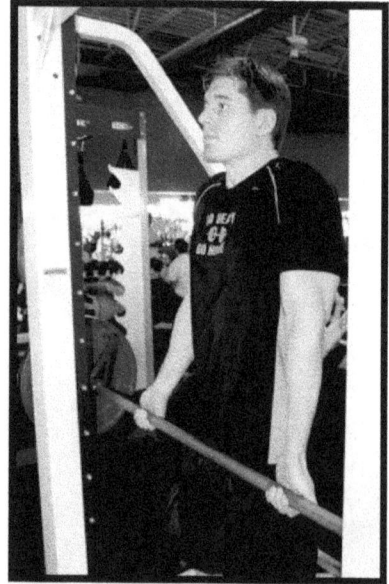

- 4 x 22-11 Upright Rows – done either with a barbell or Smith
- 4 x 11 Standing Military Press – ideally done in a press rack

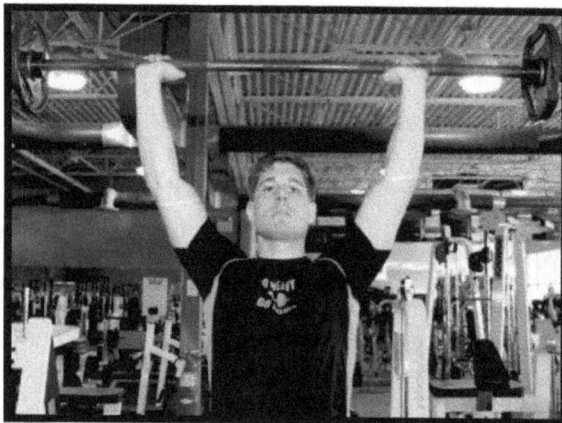

- 4 x 22-11 Barbell Rows to Chin – as described above
- 3 x 11 Side Lateral Pulls– lock the elbows and pull downward, as if coming to attention   *superset with*

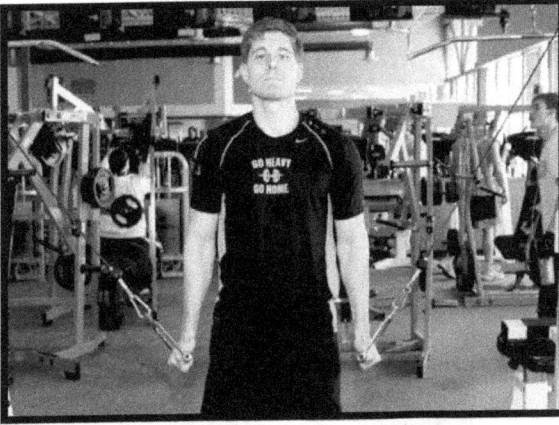

- 3 x 11 Upward Front Pulls from a low cable – hands shoulder width, pause at the top

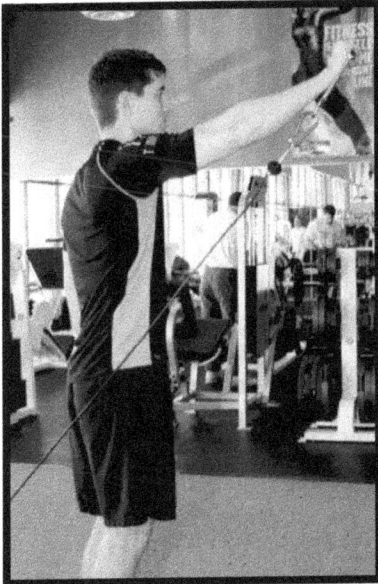

• 3 x 11 Rear Cable Cross Laterals (low) – bend at the waist, cross cables, pull out to the sides in a straight line, as if trying to touch both weight stacks while the back stays flat

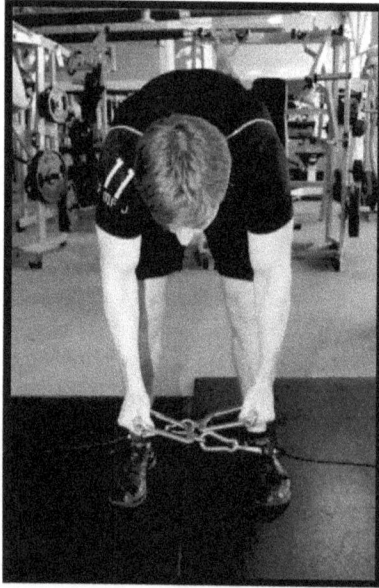

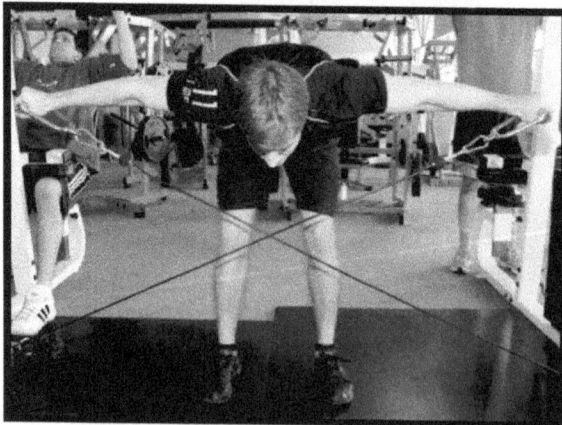

REAR CABLE CROSS LATERALS

superset with

• 3 x 11 Rear Cross-Cable Laterals (high cable) – cross cables, pull from above the forehead with arms strictly locked at elbows, down and back below the level of the shoulders

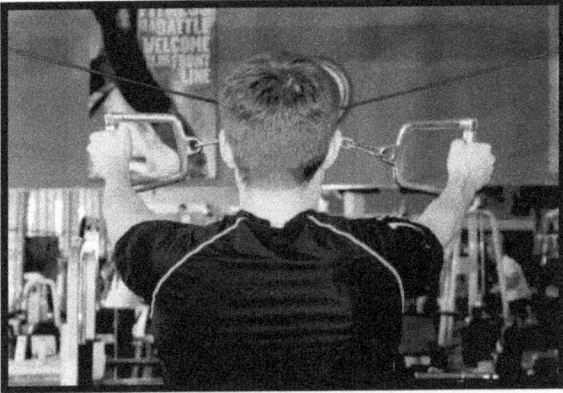

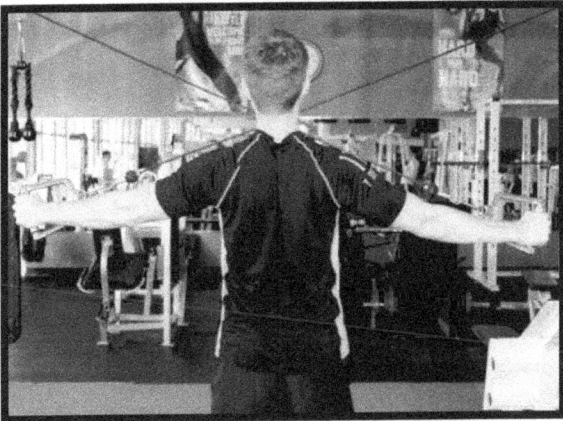

HIGH CROSS-CABLE LATERALS

#2 SHOULDERS

- 4 x 22-11 Front Shrugs
- 4 x 22-11 Rear Shrugs
- 4 x 22-11 Upright Rows
- 3 x 22 Smith Barbell Rows to Chin – done the same as the Upright rows, only on the Smith machine. The benefit to this is the straight tracking it allows.
- 4 x 11-22 Rear Military Press – wide grip, drop the bar to the top of the neck behind head

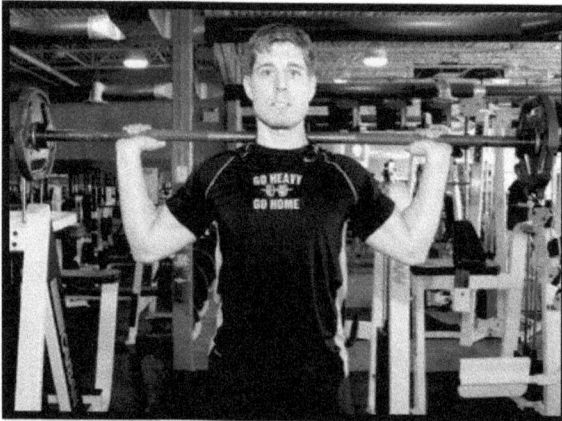

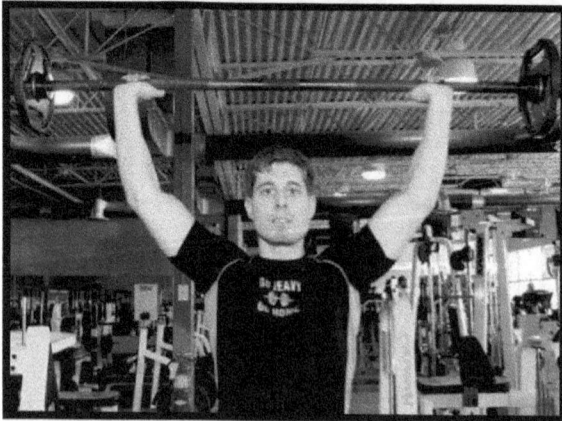

REAR MILITARY PRESS

superset with

- 4 x 22-11 Front Military press – bring the bar all the way to the collarbones on each rep

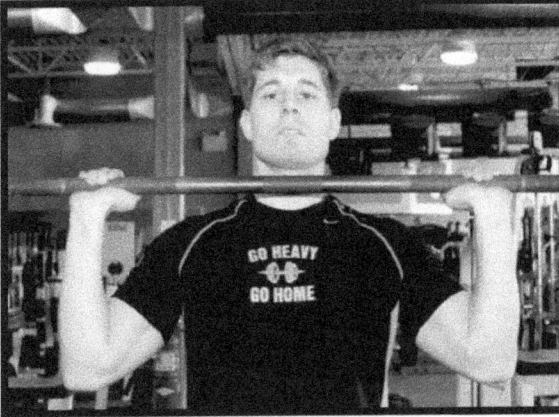

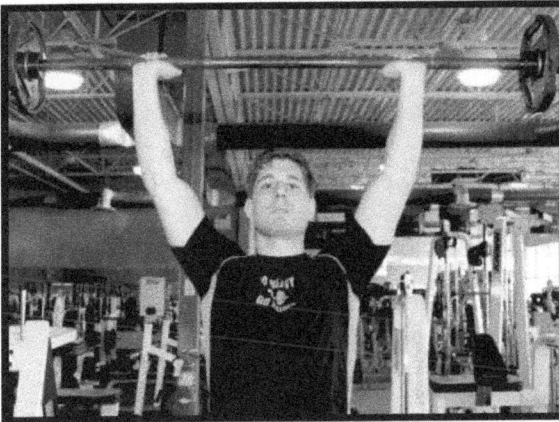

FRONT MILITARY PRESS

- 2 x 22 Seated Dumbbell Press – both hands together, press to middle directly over head   *superset with*
- 2 x 11 Alternate Standing Dumbbell Press – these are twice as heavy as the seated
- 3 x 11 Rear Single Cable Laterals – bent at the waist, pulling straight across   *superset with*
- 3 x 11 Side Cable Pulldowns – both arms simultaneously, down to the sides   *superset with*
- 3 x 11 High Handle Front Lateral Pulldowns – bring down to thighs, elbows locked

As with all Shoulder movements, you must use focus to ensure the shoulders are doing the work and not the Triceps or Biceps. This High Lateral Pulldown is to be focused on keeping the hands loose, the elbows locked and the back straight. The pull must come from the top of the shoulders, and steadily come to the top of the thighs. You will also feel this in the serratus muscles if you are executing it correctly.

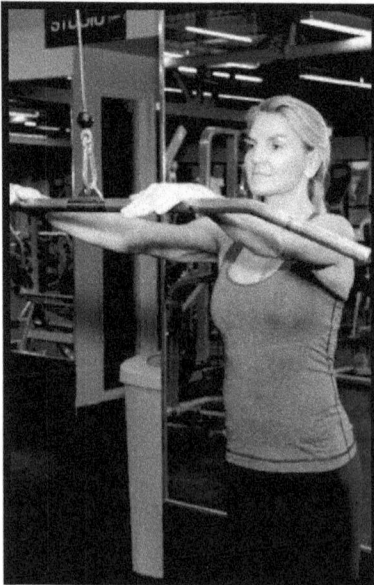

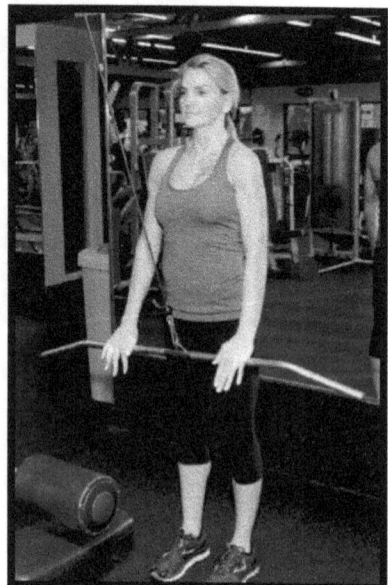

#3 SHOULDERS

- 4 x 22-11 Rear Smith Machine Press *(same as Barbell)*
- 4 x 22-11 Front Smith Machine Press
- 4 x 22-11 Standing Military Press

- 3 x 22 Barbell Rows to Chin   *superset with*
- 3 x 11 Front Barbell Lateral – raise the barbell at arms length in front of body, pause   *superset with*
- 3 x 11 Side Dumbbell Lateral - (you want to reach out to the sides rather than up or back)
- 3 x 11 Bent-over Rear Cable Laterals   *superset with*
- 3 x 11 Cross Cable Rear Laterals

- 4 x 22-11 Front then Rear Shrugs (2 Sets each)

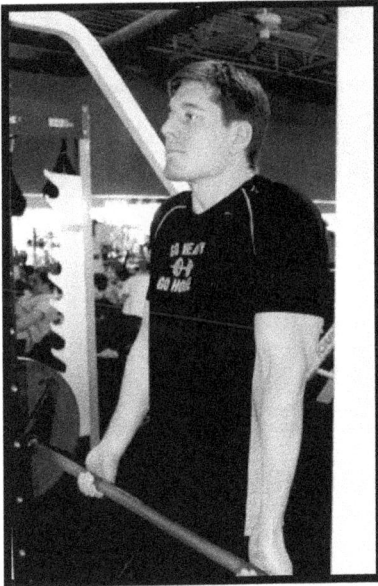 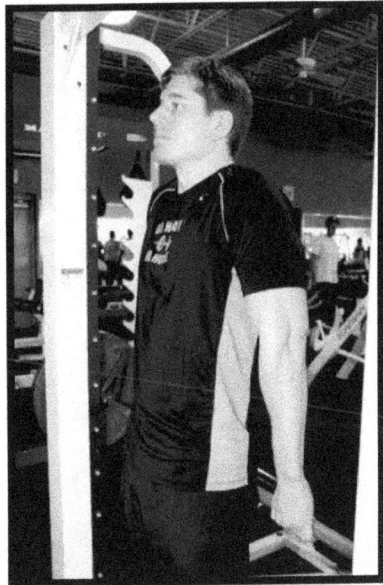

FRONT SHRUGS   *REAR SHRUGS*

#4 SHOULDERS

• 2 x 22 Smith Press Over And Back - just clear the head with these, exaggerating both the width behind and a narrow pull of the elbows on the forward part of the movement. The bar should barely clear the head in order to involve the medial deltoid as it passes from front to back. Avoid a full extension.

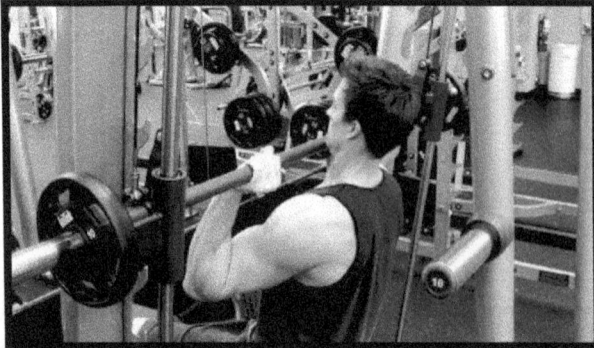

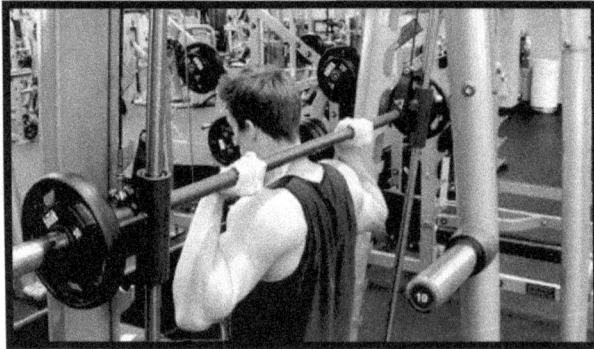

OVER AND BACK SMITH PRESS

- 2 x 22 -11 Smith Rear Press
- 2 x 22 -11 Smith Front Press
- 4 x 22-11 Upright Rows
- 4 x 22-11 Rear Barbell Rows to Chin

- 3 x 22 Alternate Dumbbell Press   *superset with*
- 3 x 22 Seated Dumbbell Press

- 3 x 11 Rear Cable Raise   *superset with*

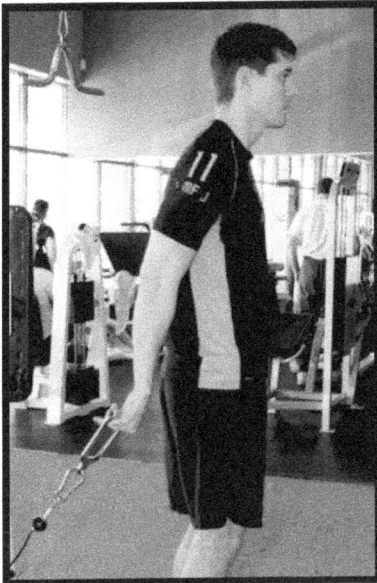

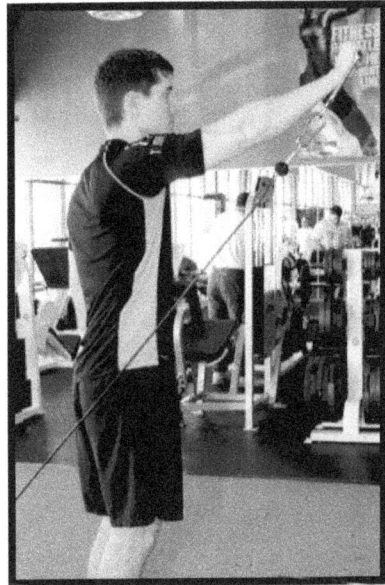

As with all shoulder movements, the hands should be loose in order to utilize the shoulder muscles and not the triceps or biceps in the pull of the cable. Start with the arm behind you and push forward toward the knuckles rather than raising the hand high.

• 3 x 11 Single Rear Lateral

This is shown with dual cables, but you would simply grasp one side at a time with the opposite hand on the knee for stability, pulling straight across from the shoulder girdle, rather than up or back, which activates the latissimus and won't fully stimulate the rear deltoids.

SINGLE REAR CABLE LATERALS

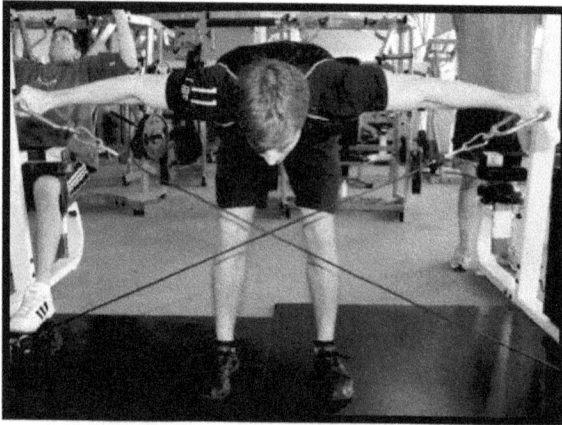

#5 SHOULDERS

- 2 x 22 Smith Over and Back – exaggerate the elbows wide behind and narrow in front

- 2 x 22 -11 Smith Rear Press
- 2 x 22 -11 Smith Front Press
- 4 x 22-11 Machine Seated Press
- 3 x 11 Front Dumbbell Laterals   *superset with*
- 3 x 11 Side Dumbbell Laterals   *superset with*
- 3 x 11 Rear Dumbbell Laterals – bent at 90°, do these with the hands facing you, rather than each other, this adds for a better pump in the middle of the rear deltoids

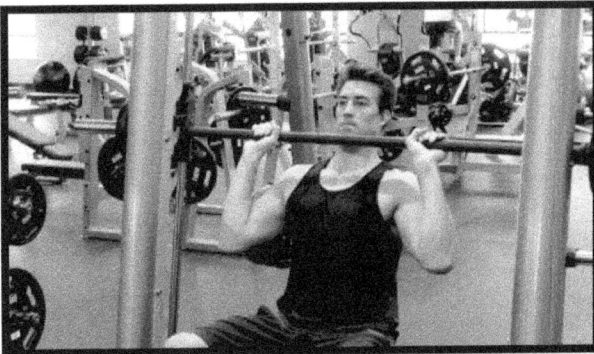

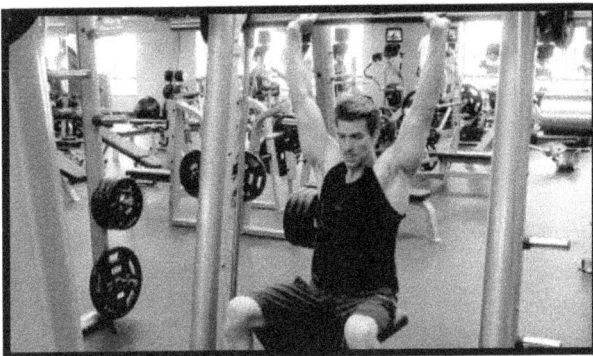

SMITH FRONT PRESS

#6 SHOULDERS

- 4 x 22-11 Military Barbell Press
- 3 x 11 Dumbbell Press - knuckles facing shoulders to begin, end facing mirror
- 4 x 22-11 Machine Press - facing IN to the machine will activate the rear deltoids first
- 4 x 22-11 Machine Press - facing OUT from the machine will activate the front deltoids
- 3 x 22 Barbell Rows to Chin

- 3 x 11 Front Dumbbell Laterals   *superset with*
- 3 x 11 Side Dumbbell Laterals   *superset with*
- 3 x 11 Rear Dumbbell Laterals

A very important point to remember when doing any type of lateral movement for the shoulders, whether with cables or with dumbbells, is to reach outward from the body, rather than trying to throw it upward with force from the back and legs. The shoulders should stay even, the elbows locked, the head up, and the legs slightly bent with just a little bounce at the 75% mark of the movement. A static hold at the top of lateral movements allows greater separation and definition between the deltoid heads, as well.

Do not mistake using lots of weight to get lots of size. The shoulders are small, tough muscles that respond with heavy compound movements, but also with slow, calibrated, isolation movements in perfect form.

#7 SHOULDERS

• 4x11 Dumbbell Presses	*superset with*
• 3x11 Front Dumbbell Laterals	*superset with*
• 3x11 Side Dumbbell Laterals	*superset with*
• 3x11 Rear Dumbbell Laterals	

• 4 x 22-11 Side Cable Laterals

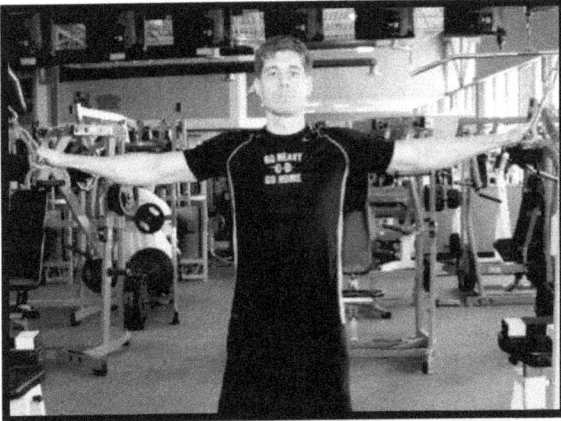

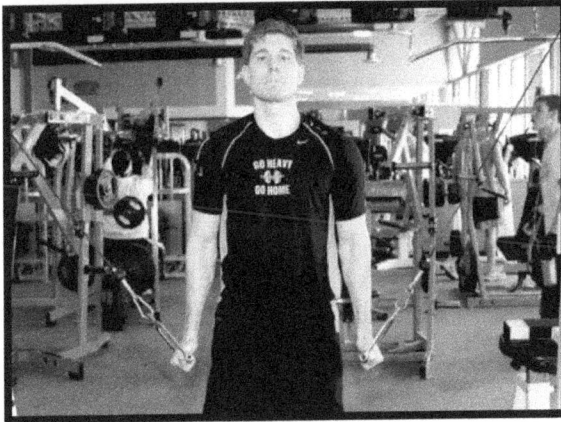

SIDE CABLE LATERALS

- 4 x 22-11 Press Machine - facing in
- 4 x 22-11 Press Machine - facing out
- 4 x 22-11 Front Cable laterals
- 4 x 22-11 Shrugs on Smith – two forward, two behind

#8 SHOULDERS

- 4 x 22-11 Barbell Shrug
- 4 x 22-11 Upright Rows

3 x 22 Alternate Front Dumbbell Raise   *superset with*
3 x 11 Bent-over Rear Dumbbell Lateral Raise

4 x 11 Dumbbell Press   *superset with*
3 x 22 Rear Cable Crossovers

#9 SHOULDERS

- 11-22-33 Shrugs Back to Bar
- 11-22-33 Shrugs Facing Bar
- 4 x 22-11 Upright Rows
- 4 x 11 Machine Press - facing in
- 4 x 11 Military Press Standing
- 4 x 22-11 Barbell Rows to Chin

3 x 11 Rear Cable Laterals   *superset with*
3 x 11 Front Cable Pulls - upward, from a low cable

#10 SHOULDERS

- 4 x 22-11 Front Shrugs
- 4 x 22-11 Rear Shrugs
- 4 x 22-11 Upright rows
- 3 x 22 Smith Rows to Chin

4 x 22-11 Rear Military press   *superset with*
4 x 11-22 Front Military Press

3 x 22 Seated Dumbbell Press   *superset with*
3 x 22 Alternating Standing Dumbbell Press

3 x 11 Rear Cross-cable Laterals   *superset with*
3 x 11 Side Cable Laterals - downward   *superset with*
3 x 11 Low Handle Side Laterals – upward   *superset with*
3 x 11 Single Handle Front Lateral Pulldowns

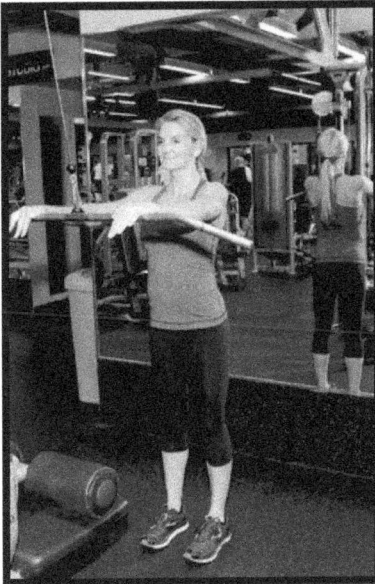

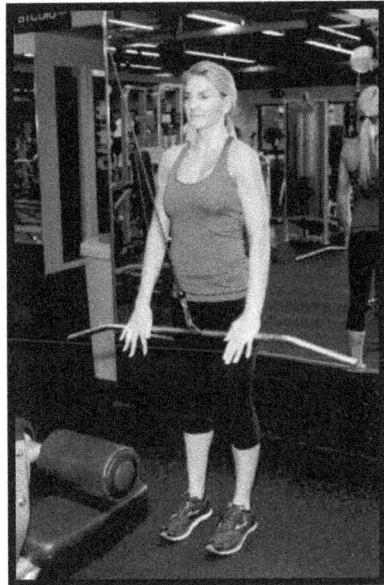

FRONT LATERAL PULLDOWNS

173

#11 SHOULDERS

- 4 x 22-11 Rear Smith Press
- 4 x 22-11 Front Smith Press
- 4 x 22-11 Machine Press
- 3 x 22 Rear Barbell Lateral   *superset with*
- 3 x 11 Front Barbell Lateral   *superset with*
- 3 x 11 Side Dumbbell Lateral

- 3 x 11 Bent-over Cable Laterals   *superset with*

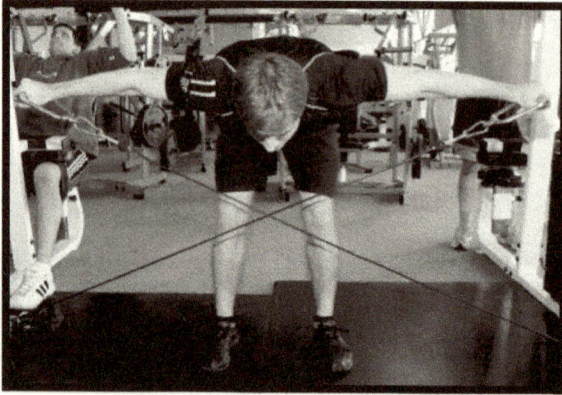

BENT OVER CABLE LATERALS

- 3 x 11 Cross-cable Laterals
- 4 x 22-11 Front Shrugs   *superset with*
- 4 x 22-11 Rear Shrugs

SHOCK AND AWE - *TRICEPS*

Many of these have the same or similar exercises, but the order and number are what's important to getting the most out of **Shock And Awe** on single bodypart workouts. The extra benefit about taking any one of these workouts and pairing them with any other bodypart, without doing compensating muscle groups, is the superior pump again to both muscle groups. This way you can pair a high priority bodypart with a low priority one and both will be fully activated.

Many people don't understand that the depth of the Triceps development comes from hitting it at many angles, with full range of motion and enough weight to instill growth, but not too much to compromise the movement. You are much better off developing all the heads equally than to continue working on the outer or long heads to gain pure size. A well defined arm looks bigger than a big fat chunk of thickness. Even my grandmother had 22 inch arms, but they were not cut and ripped!

All of these workouts concentrate on hitting all three heads of the muscle group, to add that depth without bulk. Most women want well developed arms, that cause stares and questions, but they don't need or usually want great size.

Doing too few sets is as much a mistake as overtraining. In order to get good arms, you must have good workouts, 99% of the time. You can slip and have a bad day once in a while, but your arms respond by working often, on many planes of movement, with varied handgrips and weights; never too heavy, or too light.

Apply these simple principles to all your training, every bodypart, and you will have no weaknesses. Now get to the gym.

1 TRICEPS

•4 x 22-11 Close Grip Bench Press – hands as close as comfortable, thumbs under bar, let elbows flare to sides. This movement is the ultimate Triceps size builder due to its activation of all three triceps heads. This should be first in a Triceps workout.

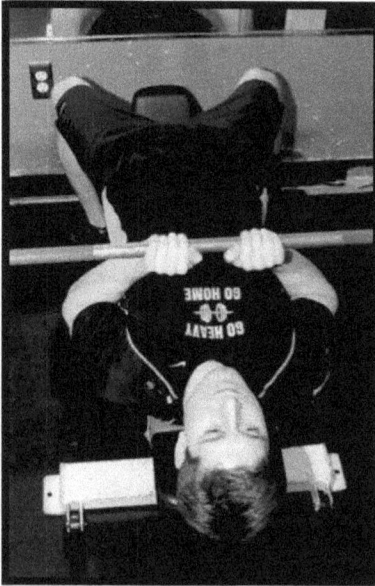

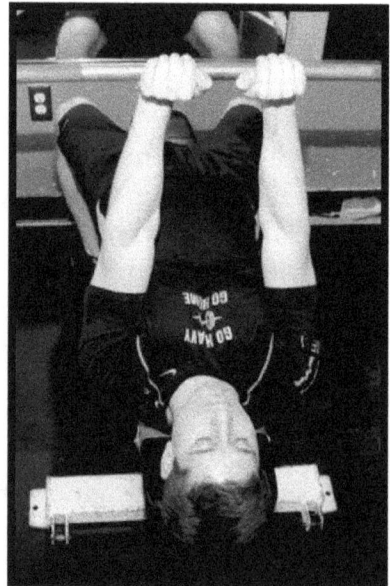

CLOSE GRIP BENCH PRESS

•4 x 22-11 Overhead Triceps Rope Pulls – elbows in and high, pushing straight forward.

This Overhead Triceps Rope Pull movement activates the long, inner head of the triceps, from elbow to armpit; so it should be done very strictly, with elbows facing forward. Do not pull down. Pull straight ahead. Doing it this way will give a full, long look to the triceps. If the rope is hitting you in the

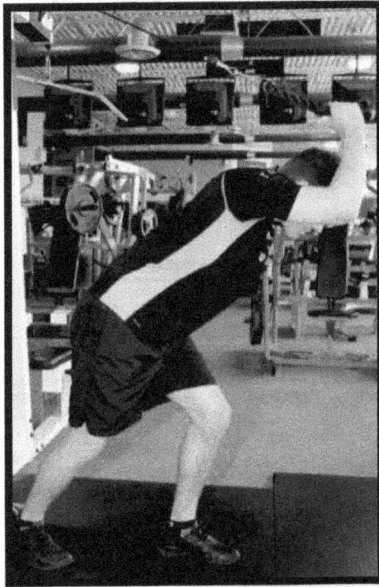

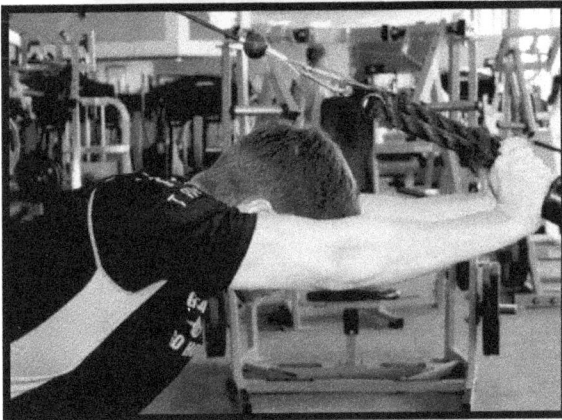

back of the head, your elbows are too low and/or your head too high. This is also a crucial core developer. Staying strict to form will work the core from top to bottom.

•3 x 22 Triceps Pushdowns – back straight, chin up, shoulders down and back, arms 90°

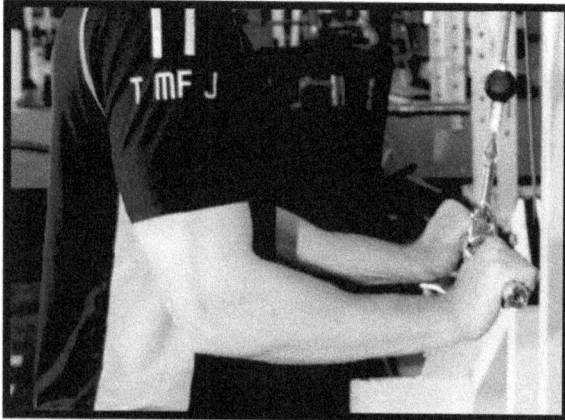

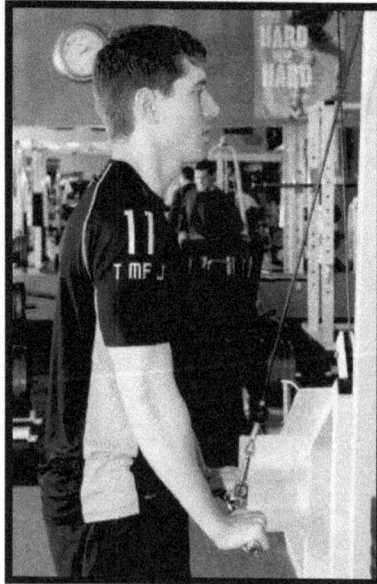

•3 x 22 Triceps Rope Pulldowns – keep hands together on rope, ***do not*** pull to sides; roll wrists to tops of hands, but keep them forced together for lower, inner triceps.

This is a finishing exercise, which gives the inner triceps full development and definition, equal to the outer head. These

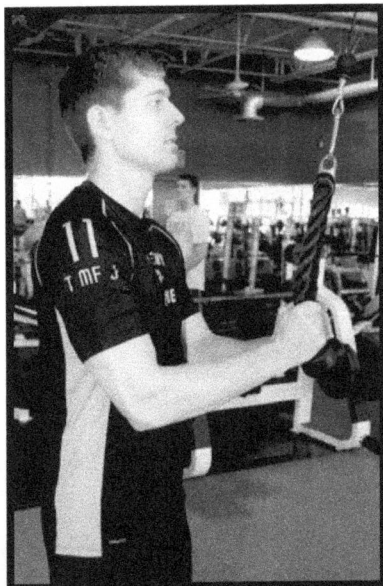

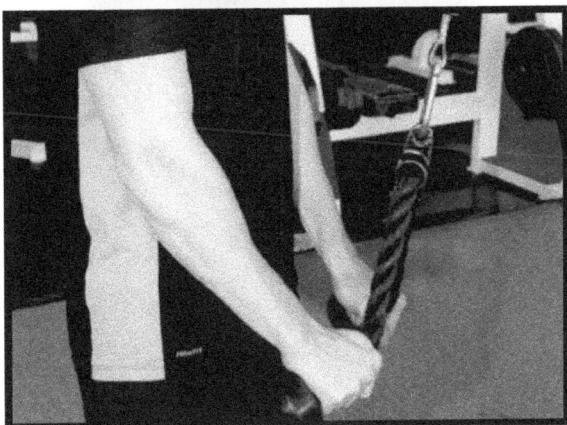

take great concentration to get them right and should be done at the end of the Triceps workout due to their light weight and specific focus.

Notice that the shoulders stay up and back, and the elbows close to the body and down, in every one of these Triceps movements. If you are leaning over the weight, you are working the trapezius. If you are raising the elbows, you are engaging the shoulders. You will not gain full Triceps development if you cheat with these other styles of execution.

#2 TRICEPS

- 4 x 22 -11 Close Grip Bench Press
- 4 x 22 -11 Overhead Rope Pulls
- 3 x 22 Triceps Rope Pulldowns

#3 TRICEPS

3 x 22 Close Grip Bench Press
4 x 11 Overhead Triceps Rope Pulls – Heavy

3 x 22-11 Triceps Pushdowns   *superset with*
3 x 11-22 Triceps Rope Pulls

#4 TRICEPS

- 4 x 22-11 Close Grip Bench Press   *superset with*
- 4 x 11 Overhead Ropes   *superset with*
- 3 x 22 Pushdowns

#5 TRICEPS

- 4 x 22-11 Close Grip Benches

- 3 x 22 Triceps Pressdowns   *superset with*
- 4 x 11 Overhead Rope Pulls Heavy

#6 TRICEPS

4 x 22-11 Decline Skull Crushers   *superset with*

3 x 22 Dips

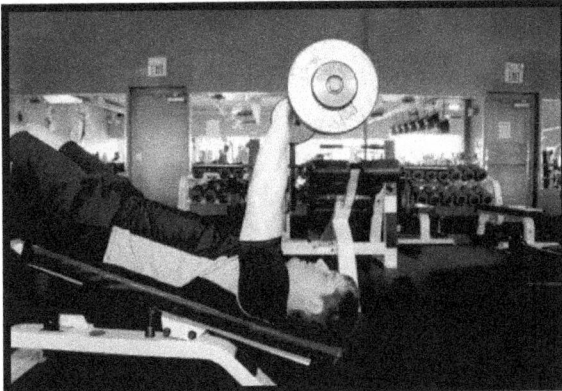

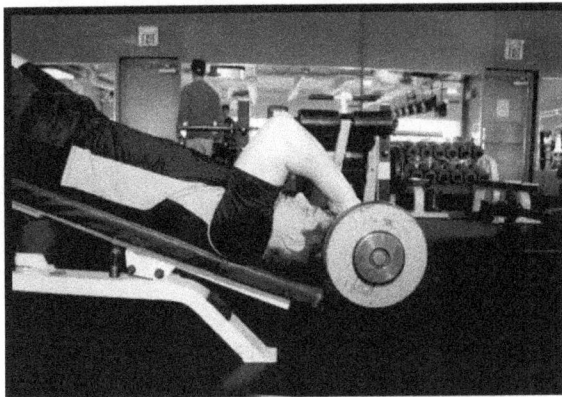

Dips, *(found in the Chest section)* can be done for both the Chest and the Triceps; the difference in the execution would be to bring the head forward and pull the legs back for Chest; and to hold the head straight up with the legs straight down or forward to put maximum emphasis on the Triceps. You would also hold a wider grip on the V-Handle of a Dip Bar for the Triceps, going narrower and further forward for the chest.

•4 x 11 Single Handle Reverse Triceps
•4 x 11 Heavy Close Grip Benches

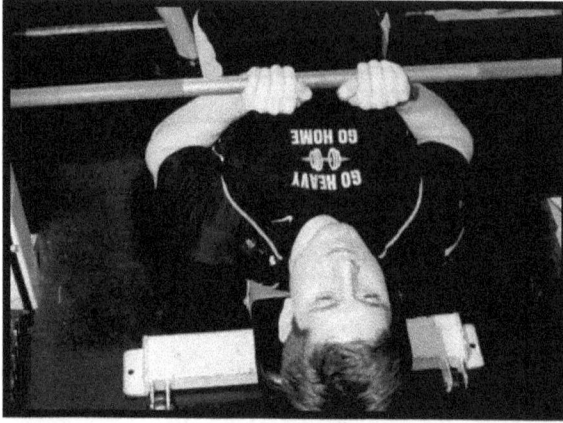

#7 TRICEPS

•4 x 22-11 Decline Skull Crushers   *superset with*
•3 x 22 Dips

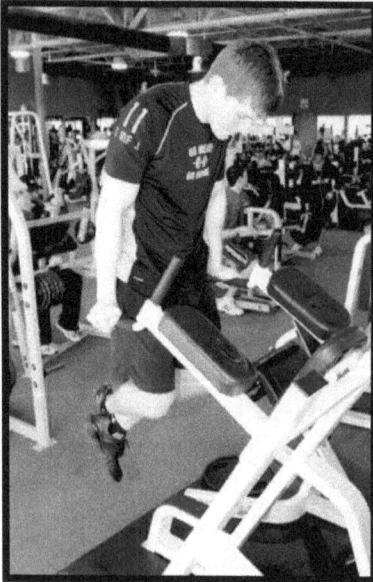

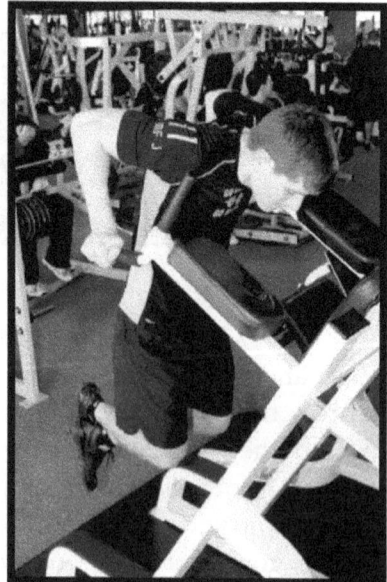

•4 x 22-11 Overhead Rope Triceps
•4 x 11 Reverse Single Handle Triceps Pulldowns
•4 x 11 Heavy Close-grip Benches

#8 TRICEPS

•33, 22, 11, 11, 22, 33 Close Grip Bench Press
•33, 22, 11, 11, 22, 33 Triceps Cable Pushdowns

#9 TRICEPS

•4 x 22-11 Close Grip Triceps Press
•4 x 22-11 Triceps Overhead Rope Pulls
•3 x 22 Triceps Pushdowns

#10 TRICEPS

•4 x 22-11 Overhead Rope Pulls
•4 x 22-11 Close Grip Benches
•4 x 22-11 Pushdowns

#11 TRICEPS

•4 x 11 French Press – this is not one of my favorites simply because the elbows flare
•4 x 22 Single Dumbbell Press – in a straight line, to top of shoulder, elbow straight up

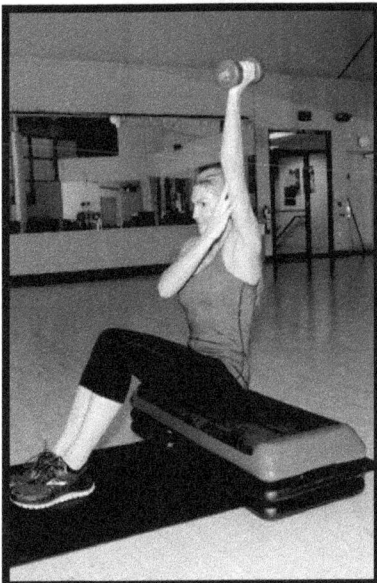

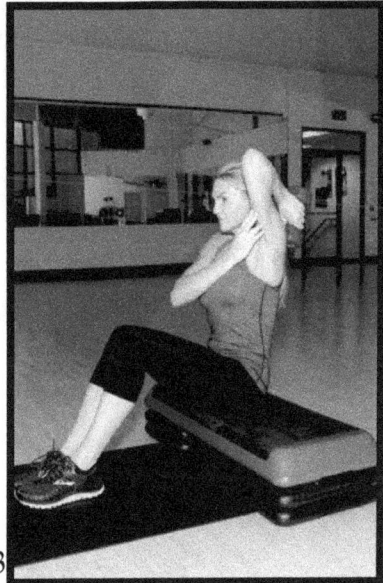

•3 x 22 Pushdowns   *superset with*

•3 x 11 Bench Dips

These can be done off a riser, a chair, a bench, a couch, whatever is available. For women who want to have a tight, defined set of Triceps, this exercise is paramount to achieving them. It is important to raise the hips at the top of the movement to activate the long head of the Triceps fully, all the way to the rear shoulder tie-in.

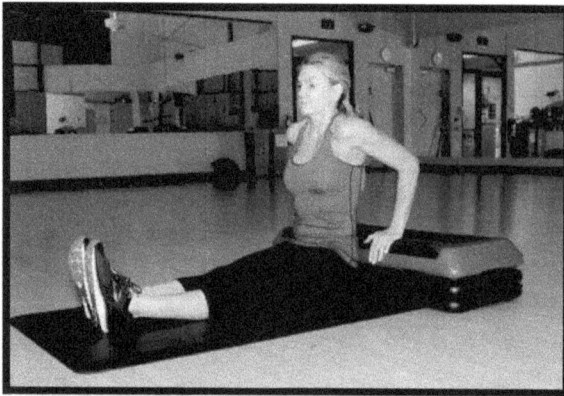

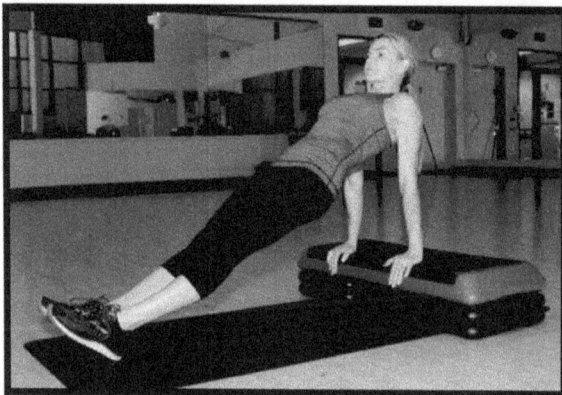

BENCH DIPS

AFTERWORD

Thank you for trying out this Shock And Awe System of working out. This will save you hours of gym time and make great shortcuts to fantastic gains in your training. It has worked for many types of physiques, from novice teenagers to seasoned gym rats and professional bodybuilders, figure, physique and bikini competitors. It has also worked well with the busy executive who values time over socializing.

It is a safe way to train because so much emphasis is put on form rather than trying to lift more weight than your body is capable of. The methods that run you through on a clock, doing as much weight as fast as possible or as many reps for totals in a given time are not only dangerous in the short term, they cause long lasting, repetitive stress injuries due to improper execution of movements, i.e.. quantity over quality.

Check out the SHOCK AND AWE MUSCLE site and leave your comments and considerations for further improvements. Leave a comment or testimonial or upload your own video to share.

I am sincerely interested in your personal progress and results, so check in often and see how others are doing as well.

My mission is to help others achieve their personal best in regard to making their body as balanced, strong and proportionate as possible. This Shock And Awe Muscle System is the way I've been able to stay injury-free and ripped at the age of 58. I've used it on myself and others for 11 plus years.

And last, remember, this is simply *A SYSTEM*, not *THE ONLY WAY TO TRAIN*. It has worked for many men, women, teens, and teams.

www.ingramcontent.com/pod-product-compliance
Lightning Source LLC
Chambersburg PA
CBHW022107280326
41933CB00007B/290